T3-BVW-027

MAKING
LOVE
AGAIN

Regaining Sexual Potency
Through the
New Injection Treatment

MAKING
LOVE
AGAIN

Regaining Sexual Potency Through the New Injection Treatment

J. Francois Eid, M.D.
Director, Erectile Dysfunction Unit
The New York Hospital-Cornell Medical Center

Carol A. Pearce

BRUNNER/MAZEL *Publishers* • NEW YORK

Library of Congress Cataloging-in-Publication Data

Eid, J. Francois.
    Making love again : regaining sexual potency through the new
injection treatment / J. Francois Eid, Carol A. Pearce.
        p. cm.
    Includes bibliographical references and index.
    ISBN 0-87630-722-5
    1. Impotence—Chemotherapy. I. Pearce, Carol A. II. Title.
RC889.E34   1993
616.6'92061—dc20   93-5918
                                                          CIP

Copyright © 1993 by J. Francois Eid and Carol A. Pearce
All rights reserved. No part of this book may be
reproduced by any process whatsoever without
the written permission of the copyright owners.

Published by
BRUNNER/MAZEL, INC.
19 Union Square West
New York, New York 10003

Manufactured in the United States of America

10 9 8 7 6 5 4 3 2

Contents

Foreword by Helen Singer Kaplan, M.D., Ph.D. .... **ix**

1. The Good News **1**
   How to Use This Book Effectively 7

2. An Overview **11**
   A Case of Diabetes.. 13
   The Background on Injections................................ 17

3. The Courage to Change.. **19**
   A Man's Reluctance 19
   Are You Ever Too Old? 22
   Going on After You've Given Up............................. 24

4. A Case of Aging **29**
   Breaking the Boundaries.................................... 29
   A Case History of Aging.................................... 30

5. How an Erection Happens **33**

6. The Causes of Erection Problems **39**
   Blockage of the Arteries................................... 40
   Drugs.. 41
   Smoking.. 42
   Alcohol.. 42
   Peyronie's Disease... 43
   Surgery.. 43
   Aging.. 43
   Injuries... 44
   Diseases 44
   Hormones... 45
   *Vein Problems (Ability to Trap Blood in
      the Penis)* 47

Tumors 47
Radiation 48
Nerves 48
Warning Signals 50

7. The Drugs: Background **53**
   The Drugs Used 55

8. Workup for Potency **59**
   History Taking 59
   The Physical Exam 66
   The Combined Injection and
       Stimulation Test 66

9. Further Testing and Followups **73**
   Second Visit 73
   Further Testing 75

10. Why Injection Therapy **83**
    Choosing an Option 83
    Use of the Injections 86
    Common Worries 88

11. How to Self-Inject **95**
    Injection Step by Step 98

12. Three Cases of Injection Therapy **105**

13. Romance **111**
    Women's Reactions to Injections 112
    What to Expect from Sexual Life
        with Injections 114

14. Questions and Answers About
    Injections and the Medications **115**

15. Prevention of Potency Problems **129**
    High-Fat Diet and High
        Serum-Cholesterol Levels 129
    High Blood Pressure 130
    Overweight 130
    Care of the Penis 131

16. Breakthroughs Ahead **133**
    Oral Medications 133
    Patches 134
    Nitric Oxide 135
    Angioplasty 137
    Medications 138

17. Conclusion **141**

    Appendix A: Self Quiz **143**

    Appendix B: Further Reading **153**

    Appendix C: Centers for Pharmacological
       Treatment of Erectile Dysfunction **155**

    Appendix D: Support Groups **159**

    Index **161**

Foreword

Helen Singer Kaplan, M.D., Ph.D.

I have had the privilege of sharing the care of many patients with Dr. Eid, and I have found him to be a rare physician in his openness to sexuality, his flexibility in treatment, and his unfailing delight when helping a man improve the quality of his sex life. These encouraging and positive therapeutic attitudes shine through the pages of this informative book on the new penile injection treatment for impotence.

Dr. Eid's book provides detailed, accurate, and up-to-date medical information about the exciting new penile injection treatment that can enable many impotent men to attain erections that look and feel normal. The text, written in simple language, free of scientific jargon, "demystifies" and explains the procedure in practical, understandable terms.

Men with physical erectile problems have several alternatives. They can give up sex, but this is a poor idea because in most cases the premature loss of sexuality is depressing and demoralizing to the man and also to his wife. Another option that some couples favor is learning to enjoy forms of lovemaking without penetration, such as oral and manual sex.

This can work very well providing both partners are satisfied with this form of stimulation. But for those men who wish to regain their ability to have erections and for those couples who want to have intercourse again, the new penile injections provide an excellent and attractive alternative to implant surgery, especially now that questions about the long-term safety of silicone penile implants have been raised.

Some psychologically minded therapists have expressed negative attitudes about penile injection treatment because they regard this as "too mechanical." Why then am I, a psychiatrist, psychoanalyst, and sex therapist so supportive of this method? It is because I have seen so many excellent results in men who were physically impotent because of diabetes, cancer surgery, or the side effects of medications being taken for various physical problems, and I have seen so much joy in couples who were able to resume their sex lives with the help of this wonderful new technology.

In my experience, injection therapy is not limited to men with the physical problems just mentioned. I have found that temporary use of injection treatment can be useful in helping patients who have *psychogenic* erectile dysfunctions to overcome their performance anxiety and gain the sexual confidence they need to resume a normal sex life. This works best when injections are combined with psychological therapy that helps the patient gain insight into his deeper problems.

Of course, penile injections are not a substitute for psychological treatment for men with psychological impotence, nor are they suitable for everyone. Injections should not be used in the attempt to override deeper and more serious psychological conflicts, and they are definitely not a cure for a lack of sexual desire for the partner. Problems with sexual guilt, intimacy, sexual desire and marital relations require expert psychological help. However, this does not detract from the fact the injections can be very helpful when the feelings are there, but the penis cannot or will not cooperate.

It is important to note that the physician's attitude towards the patient and towards sex is an important ingredient in the success of this treatment. I have seen many "horror stories" in my practice when that ingredient had been missing.

For example, I have seen patients of urologists who give a test injection dose in their office and, when a good erection develops, urge the men to "rush home" and have intercourse (with their often unprepared and startled partners) as quickly as possible, before the erection abates!

One couple was so traumatized by this type of insensitivity that they avoided sex for a year. They finally consulted me, hoping that their problem was psychological. It was not. The man was a diabetic. But the couple was soon having good sex again in response to a combination of counseling with a sex therapist and the excellent erections provided by injections, which were dispensed by Dr. Eid with proper regard to the couple's feelings.

Dr. Eid's sensitivity to the emotional needs of his patients is reflected in his method of introducing patients to injection therapy.

He administers test injections in the privacy of his office where he has the opportunity to observe the physical and emotional responses of his patients, and to adjust the dose of the medication so that it does not result in a potentially harmful prolonged erection. Only after Dr. Eid is satisfied that all is well is the patient given medication for home use in order to make love to his partner. In addition, if there are any indications that the patient has a psychological block about using the injections, or that his partner has negative feelings, Dr. Eid does not hesitate to team up with a sex therapist colleague to resolve the couple's problems and help them towards a better sex life.

If after reading this book you think that injections could be the answer to your sexual problem, it is important for you to choose a doctor who has special interest, skill, and experience in sexual medicine. This might be a medical sex therapist who can evaluate whether the injections are emotionally and physically right for you and your partner and can help you learn to use the injections in an optimal way. Or else it can be a urologist like Dr. Eid who has special skills and experience in the treatment of impotence arising from physical causes. It is important that you steer away from urologists and therapists who are not specialists in this type of treatment.

Injection treatment is a great technological breakthrough that offers an attractive treatment option for men with different types of erectile difficulties. However, this is an emotionally potent procedure and the best results are obtained when injections are administered by a professional who is sensitive to the emotional meaning of the patient's sexual problem and of this treatment, and—above all—has the skills and sensitivity to enlist the cooperation of the partner. This is critical to the ultimate success of all treatments for impotence, for even if the patient attains excellent erections through injections, his sex life will not improve unless his partner is also gratified and pleased.

I think it is a tribute to Dr. Eid's keen awareness of these important emotional issues that he has asked me, a woman and a psychiatrist, to write this introduction to his excellent book on the new injection treatment for impotence.

MAKING
LOVE
AGAIN

Regaining Sexual Potency
Through the
New Injection Treatment

1

The Good News

Male sexual potency is essential to life itself. Being able to get a fully rigid and lasting erection is far more important to a man's sense of self-worth and well-being than most women can ever imagine. The ability to function sexually is inextricably linked with the way a man sees himself and his role in the world. That is why men undergo an experience of nightmare proportions when erections falter or disappear.

It's amazing the things men tell me, and it's sad to see how much in pain some men are today—in the 1990s! I have met men in their 40s who have never made love and never told anybody before they told me. They think about sex every second of the day, and every time a woman speaks to them they go into a kind of state of shock.

Until some 10 years ago, very little could be done to alleviate male potency problems. Now the news is nothing but good. The new self-injection therapy is giving a viable option to men with potency disturbances due to a variety of causes, including disease or aging. It has been discovered that several drugs, on practically painless injection into the penis, can safely create an erection strong enough for penetration, lasting 30 minutes or more.

However, if you are like most people, your knowledge about erection problems has not kept pace with the times. Consider these facts:

1. At least 10 million and possibly as many as 20 million men in America suffer from varying degrees of impotence stemming from *physical* causes.
2. Up until the 1980s, impotence was regarded as a mental problem. Even such renowned sex experts as Masters and Johnson concluded that it's all in your head. Now, with a greater understanding of erectile dysfunction, the medical community has reversed its stand, concluding that impotence is *physical*—not psychological—in more than 80% of all cases.
3. Until only a decade ago, most doctors despaired of ever being able to provide any option for potency problems except a surgical implant—a prosthesis. Then, in the 1980s, the drugs papaverine, phentolamine, and prostaglandin E1 (PGE$_1$) were discovered to be capable of producing safe, trouble-free erections when injected into the penis. This new method of injecting medication that combats erectile dysfunction is self-administered at home.
4. The injection treatment with these drugs represents a revolutionary breakthrough in the treatment of erectile failure. Since the discovery of their effects, these drugs, as well as psychosexual therapy, have enjoyed wide use in the new specialized area of urology known as Erectile Dysfunction (ED).

This book explores injection therapy in depth, from diagnosis to learning and becoming comfortable with self-administration. Step by step, you will learn what to expect in the first visit to a dysfunction specialist, how to self-inject, what the drugs are, how they work, what their potential side-effects are, how to ease this therapy into your sexual life, and what the future holds for treatment for this very common and troubling ailment.

What's stopping you? If you're like most men, you may entertain some erroneous ideas when it comes to potency, and this causes you to give up in the face of impotence. You may think you're too old and that sex is something for the young. Maybe you have convinced yourself that you're just not as virile as you once were, or that something is going on in your head that you simply don't understand. In any event, you may have convinced yourself that you just don't care anyway. Case closed.

Your partner, meanwhile, still feels sexual desire and keenly suffers from the loss of physical closeness. This is something men often forget: Women struggle with fears about loss of attractiveness as the reason for their husband's faltering potency. These fears can be especially devastating as a woman ages and worries about losing her looks.

If this is the case with you and your spouse, perhaps you'll get some comfort from the fact that even many practicing physicians haven't heard about how effective the self-injection treatment is today. A great number of doctors still remain unaware of the remarkable results being achieved via injection therapy. Is it any wonder, then, that the news has still reached so few of the people who could benefit the most?

Unfortunately, if you, or a man you know, does manage to brave the embarrassment of asking a family doctor for help, you may meet with a lack of understanding that reinforces despair and resignation. The resulting assault on the ego is as unnecessary as it is painful. Such frustration is needless because the news is really very good: Today, erectile dysfunction can be successfully treated.

Keep in mind: The world of medicine offers safe, effective drugs that do produce erections. This self-injection treatment of these medications into the penis shortly before intercourse produces erections and is so simple that men who discover the medications find it hard to believe their good fortune.

One warning: The purpose of this book is not to replace a visit to the doctor, urologist, or specialist, but rather to offer a guide to what is available, information not likely to be found accurately anywhere else. Only physicians can prescribe the drugs and injections.

This information starts and ends with this fact: Most men who suffer from erectile dysfunction (ED) should be on injection treatment with one of the new and safe drugs, at least initially. Treatment works in the majority of patients, and in the next five years, will most certainly be considered the gold standard treatment for erectile dysfunction. Everything else will be secondary.

At the same time, the underlying thrust of this book is to take the fear out of impotence treatment. Having established an ongoing and rapidly growing Pharmacological Erection Program (PEP) at The New York Hospital–Cornell Medical Center in New York City, I see the same excitement over and over from my patients when they encounter this good news.

Some men are moved to tears when they confide in me about this problem, which may have been gnawing at them for years. And then they are even more moved when the problem is alleviated in a short time. To know that medical experts do exist who take their problems seriously is also something that touches them deeply. The overwhelming number of responses from my radio and TV talks demonstrates that the general population wants to know more about these potency treatments, an indication to me of how far-reaching the effects of erectile dysfunction are.

Here is a typical scenario from our Erectile Dysfunction Unit: Mr. G was 64 years old, a smoker who had undergone coronary artery bypass surgery (so there was atherosclerosis). He used to drink heavily, but quit. He had been married for 30 years and had an excellent relationship with his wife—except for a problem with erections. His erections started weakening five years before he came to this Unit. This is typical of how long men may wait before seeking treatment, often because of shame but usually because they haven't been aware that this is a medical problem that can be successfully treated.

In the form we have all new patients fill out, we ask: Is your partner interested in having your sexual problem treated? Mr. G wrote: "You're damned right!" He was quite a fellow.

He rated his infrequent erections as 30% of normal, which means just a fullness of the penis. He hadn't been able to penetrate for at least four years. While he continued to have ejaculation, he rarely experienced orgasm with an erect penis.

Mr. G told us that he started consulting doctors in 1985. They tested his penile pulses. (We find that when this test reads normal, 50% of the time it is actually abnormal. Doctors used to do this test on a patient, find it was normal, and then tell him the problem was all in his head.) Then the doctors he consulted tested his testosterone level (which is always borderline/low in this man's age group), found that it was low, and gave him testosterone. Of course, his libido (sex drive) improved a bit—but not much. So he saw another doctor, who did a sleep test.

Nocturnal testing, which measures the number and strength of erections over a period of three nights, is important in people with suspected psychological problems, but it's a waste of time and money in a man of his age group because he's well adjusted and happily married but with physical risk factors. Of course, the nocturnal testing showed he had very poor erections. The problem was organic.

Then he had a nerve conduction test and a battery of blood tests to further check his testosterone. Again, the testosterone was low, but giving him testosterone would increase the size of his prostate and have a secondary effect such as increased urinary frequency. So why bother checking it? His libido was good and the night test had showed he had an organic problem. The nerve conduction showed normal—as could be expected. And so there he was, from 1985 to 1990, getting useless testosterone injections.

Finally, a diagnostic service suggested he consult our Erectile Dysfunction Unit. He brought his wife along.

Mr. G was six feet tall, a nattily dressed businessman who traveled a great deal. He described something that is very important—bad circulation and cramps in his legs. His feet were often cold and he got cramps when walking. Leriche's syndrome is a blockage of the aorta, the blood vessel, at about the umbilicus, right below the renal arteries, and it affects all the organs below the waist. Leg cramps and impotency are classic Leriche's complaints.

The only test Mr. G hadn't had yet in his medical search was a penile injection. I injected him while he was standing up looking at an erotic magazine. His response to the medication wasn't 100% terrific, but it did run between 50 and 60%, definitely an erection he could use during intercourse—and it would probably get better with stimulation. He was extremely happy with the results and came right back for the teaching session that would show him how to administer the drug injection himself, at home.

What impressed me particularly about Mr. G was that he was very relaxed. Though he had been searching for answers for five years, he hadn't given up. By the time some men see me, they're enraged or desperate, but Mr. G said nothing of that. He just came and said, "Can you do something for me?"

How to Use This Book Effectively

The text breaks down into three main parts:

1. Diagnosis and treatment. All about the medications, how they are used in diagnosis and treatment, who can benefit from them. Included are illustrative case histories of actual patients.
2. Self-diagnosis quiz to help you evaluate symptoms and get an inkling as to whether they might be psychological or physical in nature.
3. Directory of experts and resources nationwide.

To get the most out of this material, use this as a workbook. First, read to acquaint yourself with the latest information on erection problems and this new form of treatment. Use the self-diagnosis quiz to get a sense as to whether you (or your mate) suffer from a physical as opposed to a psychological problem. Then, make up your mind what you want to do.

Do you want to leave matters as they are? Are you content to do nothing? Or do you want to make a change, to reach out to improve your quality of life?

If you want to try injection pharmacotherapy, contact a urologist at a center specializing in this treatment (leading centers are listed in the back of this book) and go in for an individualized diagnosis. If you (or your mate) prove to be a suitable candidate for injection therapy, then this book can help you follow your doctor's instructions on how to perform self-injections. Step-by-step, the drawings and the explanatory text tell you everything you need to know when you're at home with the medications.

Keeping the romance alive at the same time is an important

aspect of potency and should not be forgotten in the rush to inject. It is especially important to know that age is no barrier.

When I think of aging and its effect on potency, and how
these treatments can help even against the ravages of time, I
think of Mr. A, an artist in his 80s, who came to see us after having literally given up on being sexually active. His wife had also
given up. After an injection in this unit, he developed a tremendous erection. It went down, so he was able to leave, but when he
got home, it returned. Exhausted, his wife finally sent him back
to us so he could be detumesced. (After about four to five hours,
a very rigid erection can be painful—and dangerous.) When he
came back, he bragged that he had given his wife 13 orgasms. I assumed he was talking about another time, over a period of
months, but he said he meant in the last couple of hours. I said,
are you sure? He said yes. You're not bragging? No, I'm not bragging. It's true.

It is somewhat unusual for someone in his 80s to respond so
vigorously to injections. Usually, it is only patients with a *psychogenic* problem (rather than a *physical* problem) who develop prolonged erections. In these patients, an antidote is always given to
bring down the erection before they leave the office.

When I'm in a social situation, if I'm pressed to tell people
my specialty, some act very amused. Sometimes, people laugh
nervously. Some people are puzzled, maybe shocked or embarrassed. Usually, the ones who are shocked will recover to ask
questions, serious questions, and then ease up as I talk because I
discuss potency in an easy, natural way. That is how I feel about
it. Then, other people adopt that attitude after a few seconds.
Some people take a little longer than others. Some people laugh
every time they see me. But, in general, people want to hear all
they can.

I find it especially interesting that there is a lot of curiosity
from women. Women are fascinated about men's obsession with

erections. They love to hear that men want to remain sexually active with aging, and to hear about men who have erections of very long duration. Actually, the difference between men's and women's attitudes toward potency stands out vividly in my practice. But they come together on one key point: They want making love to be like it used to be—when they were 18 or 20. And now, with injection therapy, it can be. In this way, you and your sexual partner can create your own new beginning.

2

An Overview

So many exciting changes are taking place in the world around us today that make this book and this new treatment possible.

Society is opening up, talking freely about sexual problems including those with erections. Men are coming to seek treatment who were not seeking treatment before. Now they see that renewed potency is possible.

There is new treatment for prostate cancer—radical prostatectomy—that is curing men with cancer. At the same time, this can create potency problems. Now we have an easy pharmacological treatment for patients who have potency problems arising from extirpative cancer surgery. Major institutions such as Memorial Sloan-Kettering Cancer Center find that patients want not only to have their cancer taken care of, but also to retain quality of life. They want to be sexually active.

Men are living longer, they are remarrying. Couples stay sexually active longer than ever before. People are recognizing that it's not necessary to give up the sexual pleasures of youth just because they are getting older. People are retiring sooner, to enjoy quality of life. Therefore, they have more time to be at home spending time together. Suddenly, erections are not there any-more, and their enjoyable life seems to be destroyed.

Take Mr. W. He came to us in his 60s with a history of both hypertension and prostate cancer. His cancer had been treated five years before with radiation seeds, and he was doing well with it, feeling fit. He was taking several medications for hyperten-sion, although he hadn't had an erection in about five years be-cause of the effects of the drugs. Then his wife died. He still had no erections, but he was depressed at his wife's death and didn't care.

A few months before he came to see us, he had met a woman in her 40s and they began to spend time together. He shortly be-came concerned about satisfying this younger woman sexually and decided to look further into his problem with erections. He was not optimistic, but still he was excited about his new rela-tionship and hoping he could do something about fulfilling it sexually. His cancer doctor referred him to us.

Actually, his response to injections was not too good—40%, at best. We generally set 60% as what's needed for penetration and most of our patients respond this well. I told Mr. W to stop smoking to get rid of one risk factor.

When we get a poor response to the medications, the first thing I wonder is if the response is poor because the patient is in a doctor's office or because his arteries are bad. I used to say, well, your arteries are severely blocked, but I learned that even though they may be blocked, a man could possibly get a good enough erection at home to penetrate. So we don't give up. I told Mr. W that this was not the end. We brought him back, taught him to self-inject and gave him samples of medication to try at home. He was hopeful and actually he did manage to get more of an erec-tion at home than he had gotten in five years.

Another reason potency treatment is becoming so popular is that potency itself is becoming demystified: Men are talking more about their erections to their wives. Women are talking to their friends about erection problems and how it affects them also. Men talk to friends about their problems with erections. Suddenly, people are recognizing that having an erection problem is like having hypertension: They don't have to be ashamed of it; it doesn't mean guilt or inadequacy. It just means they have a physical problem.

I even have one patient who injects himself from time to time even though he has no regular partner. He just wants to know that he's still potent.

Psychologists and psychiatrists are also recognizing that a lot more potency problems have a physical origin. Even when the problem is psychological, people can be helped more readily when the problem is addressed physically.

Finally, doctors are recognizing that potency treatment is important for their patients and are actually beginning to *ask* their patients if they have problems with erections.

At the same time, we are experiencing breakthroughs in medicine, such as in the management of diabetic patients. These people are living longer, insulin is improving, we are better able to control diabetes, so we're seeing now more long-term complications of diabetes. Erection problems are one of the complications. Now we have simple methods to improve erections for diabetics as well.

A Case of Diabetes

Mr. N, a 70-year-old widower, had difficulty attaining an erection. He had suffered from severe depression after his wife died, and he thought that was the problem. However, he married again and still his erections refused to respond. He also noted that at times he could have an orgasm and not feel it, which disturbed him greatly.

Mr. N had been under treatment for diabetes. When his doctor told him that his sugar was getting worse and dieting couldn't control it, he was placed on Glucotrol, an oral medication to lower blood sugar. Mr. N told his doctor about not feeling orgasms and about his faltering erections, but every time he brought up the subject, the doctor steered him into another topic. Mr. N sought out another doctor.

When he went on vacation with his new wife in Puerto Rico, he looked forward to a revived sex life. Normally, his erections were better on vacation, due to relaxation, but this time they were even worse! He rationalized that this must be because he was sexually more active and didn't have enough time to "rest" between interludes. Finally, he stopped having erections altogether.

When he finally came to see us, he told me that he had stopped hugging and holding his new wife because they would get aroused and then nothing would happen. He closed himself off from her, since getting close led only to more frustration.

He and his wife didn't discuss the matter, and he was so distraught about coming to see me, that he didn't tell her he was coming. Clearly upset, he asked: "How many times can I arouse my wife and not perform?"

In the course of one visit, this man's misery, like so many in my files, was easily resolved.

After trying injection therapy successfully, he came back to my office beaming. There was a pause, and then he said, "Dr. Eid, my wife asked me to tell you something, too."

I said, "Oh," expecting a complaint or maybe some special request.

"Yes. She said she wants *you* to know that I'm a good lover. And that she enjoys having sex with me."

The same thing is true with spinal cord injuries. Each year there are about 8,000 new spinal cord injuries in mostly young men. These men make a difference in our society. We have better rehabilitation. These patients learn how to take care of their own health, they're trained. They get jobs, they're in relationships, they remain sexually active. Even young men in their teens and twenties who suffer spinal cord injuries that render them impotent as well as immobile can be helped with the new potency treatment so that they can marry and actually have a family. To see these men regain that power—that hope—is especially moving to all of us at this Unit. Being sexually active, enjoying intimacy, goes with being human. Sexual union satisfies and completes people deeply.

All of this constitutes an overall picture of people seeking to live full lives, a scenario that's happening in our society today all around us. It's not just one thing, it's not just the technology that's available today to treat potency. The technology is only a part of this picture.

In this new scenario, it is no longer appropriate to treat all men with erection problems the same way. That would be like treating somebody with hypertension (high blood pressure) with a diuretic only, or treating everybody with pneumonia with the same antibiotic. In the treatment of high blood pressure, we now have options such as calcium channel blockers, alpha blockers, beta blockers, and diuretics, as well as all sorts of other options. The same is true for erection problems.

The injection therapy brings a new option for men suffering from erectile dysfunction, a new possibility for a better life.

This new option is built on the concept of using medications to specifically control erections.

This is the first time that we human beings have a specific medication that *reliably* gives most men an erection. It is painless, it is easy to do, it is harmless, it is effective, it is not expensive, and patient response is tremendous. It is a medical breakthrough: a breakthrough for men in urology; a breakthrough for men in general; and a breakthrough for couples, because a woman's life is just as much affected by her partner's potency problems as the man's.

Generally, potency problems strike in a man's mid-50s to early 60s, yet a man of this age still has another 20 or more years of potential sexual activity ahead of him.

Mr. M came to me at age 59, in good health except for angina for which he had undergone a coronary artery bypass five years before. After the bypass surgery, he had problems with erections.

Some time before, he had read an article in *The Wall Street Journal* about injection therapy. Still, he typified the men who wait so long before doing something even after reading about it. He started actively seeking help only some two years before he finally came to our Unit.

The same amount of arterial disease that had existed at the level of the bypass was present in the vessels of his penile arteries. Atherosclerotic vascular disease is not just specific to the coronaries. And it had caught up with him. Or maybe it had been present to some extent before, but he was more concerned about his heart then, which took precedence.

I gave him a small test injection during his first visit and he got an erection that lasted an hour and a half. So, for five years he could have had erections like this one instead of suffering with the problem. It makes me wonder how many men have a problem now and will wait at least five years before coming for help.

Every patient who comes here tells a different story, but they usually all have more in common than they ever realize. Take Mr. D, in his 60s. He looked like an older James Bond, sophisticated, impeccably dressed. Like most widowers, he told me the poignant story of his relationship with his wife and then her death. For the last four years of her life, she was ill and he only "kissed her a lot and loved her dearly." He never went "outside the household for sex" while she was alive, but after she died, a friend recommended a prostitute and he tried the experience, excited as a little boy. It was then that he found he could not penetrate, nor could he in later attempts. Then he found a new partner whom he came to love very much.

One day on the golf course, a friend, a very earthy type, told him that later he was going to tell him a secret. Mr. D said OK. When he met his friend a week later, the friend proceeded to tell him about having three operations on his prostate because he couldn't urinate, and how then he couldn't have erections. The man had always been active and used to tell Mr. D stories about his affairs. He then told him that he was now taking injections in his penis and getting erections that lasted an hour.

Mr. D couldn't wait, he told me, to find out if his problems were similar. So he came for treatment and, to his satisfaction, found they were.

The Background on Injections

The idea of injections to produce erections was developed by accident in the early 1980s (See Chapter 7). It was not until 1985–86 that doctors advanced the concept of self-injection at home.

The initial response among physicians was cold. Doctors could not imagine a patient injecting himself in the penis. Everybody thought the penis was too sensitive, that injections would be too painful, too cumbersome, perhaps not effective, too risky. Moreover, the complications initially encountered were daunting. They included scarring of the penis and priapism (prolonged erections).

By exploring further, however, physicians learned that these complications are seldom found in appropriately treated patients. If the patient is followed medically, as for any other medical condition, complications are minimal. There are far fewer complications from these medications than from a blood thinner, for example, or an antihypertensive, or antibiotics.

At the same time, pharmacological treatment is effective in over 80% of patients. It works for men with spinal cord injuries, multiple sclerosis, circulatory problems, and other medical problems. It also works in men who have psychogenic erectile dysfunction who have not been helped by other conservative established treatment modalities.

With injection therapy, most men regain their potency in a very simple fashion without surgery. The injections don't hurt. And men often experience even better potency than they used to have when they were 30 years old. So men are really excited. They feel they are now better sexually than they used to be. They can get an erection when they want and they don't have to worry about whether or not they're going to get one. The medications work!

3

The Courage to Change

A Man's Reluctance

There are millions of men who have given up on sex because they are having erection problems. They make excuses. They say they're not interested anymore, they've got better things to do, they're getting too old, etc. It becomes a big job for a woman to counteract these excuses and convince her mate to seek treatment. It also takes a lot of courage for a man to come to see us on his own, or at someone else's urging. So many men still find it difficult to talk about the subject.

Mr. I, a 40-year-old Irish male who had emigrated from Ireland 10 years earlier, couldn't talk about his potency problem. There he was, 40 years old, and I was astounded at the amount of suffering he had experienced because he was so closed up. He claimed that when he danced with a woman, he got feelings of excitement but got no erection. Then, when he was alone, he said, he got good erections. With a woman in a sexual situation, he either didn't get an erection at all or, if he got one, he would quickly lose it before penetrating. The fact that he could get good erections when alone told me right away that his problem was most likely psychological.

He was a construction worker who liked to drink a lot of beer daily. I pointed out to him that alcohol is a depressant. It keeps you cut off, not wanting to communicate. So that made him less "present" to his sexual unhappiness. Drinking pacified him, numbed him, making it seem as if it didn't really matter. As a result, he became even more resigned. The beer drinking also suppressed his sexual desire, or libido, so that now it was more comfortable for him to give up. But his libido returned the next day when he wasn't numb anymore.

When I came up against that resignation, I told him it didn't have to be this way. I tried to get him to see that another way might be possible; I argued my best.

What happens too often is that there is a lack of intimacy that occurs for many humans in general. Intimacy, to me, means not just a sexual relationship, but being able to communicate all the little shameful thoughts about your feelings that you may not be adequate or good enough. It was almost impossible for Mr. I to just say something like that. He had suffered from his problem for at least 15 years. His pain was tremendous, but he was barely aware that he was suffering.

Suffering signs? A lot of sadness. At one point in talking to me, he was almost tearful. A lot of loneliness. Because he knew he couldn't function like other men, he avoided being with a woman. He was trapped in a very painful circle and couldn't see his way out. He had a problem and the problem became the reason he was alone. The payoff for remaining in this situation was he didn't have to face the problem.

I started by acknowledging to Mr. I the risk he took in talking to me about this—what little he was able to get out. He had taken a bold step, so I emphasized how courageous he was. Essentially, he did what Christopher Columbus did, I told him.

He set sail into the unknown, willing to gamble for the possibility of a great discovery. I told him that this is how it would be from now on. Each time he stretched out of his comfort zone to seek something else, things could become much better. There was something more to life; it didn't have to be hopeless. He listened carefully, but I knew it was hard for him to accept. I was talking against 40 years of how things had always been for him.

I know a lot of men hope their problem is physical. That strikes them as more manly. Also, then they don't have to wrestle with it. They can just take an injection and get fixed. I sent Mr. I for a sleep test, which showed normal erections. Having laid the groundwork, I sent him to a sex therapist. I also told him we would work in conjunction with the sex therapist in giving him small doses of medications so that he could avoid freezing up in a sexual situation. Most men will go to a sex therapist at that point, once we've made the tests and found no physical problem. They realize this treatment is not so bad. They realize that help exists for them. And that it is possible to be potent and have a relationship.

After several sessions with a sex therapist, Mr. I started sexual activity again, and with the help of injections, was able to have sexual relations with penetration and maintain his erection to orgasm. Both he and his partner raved over the reliability of injections. He was encouraged to attempt sexual relations without them, and on subsequent office visits, he reported that his performance anxiety had diminished considerably and that the volume of medication needed to obtain a firm erection was diminishing rapidly, indicating again that his condition was psychological in nature. On his last visit two months later, he described normal sexual activity without the assistance of penile injections. He was successfully "weaned off" injections.

Mr. I, in turn, reminded me of a patient from Oman (The

Middle East) whom we saw briefly. At one time he had been embarrassed sexually in front of a woman. Being a man from the
Middle East, he might as well have cut his throat after that
because he could never ever allow himself to be put into a
situation where that might occur again. Giving him the
medications for injections gave him the assurance he needed, the
no-risk backup he absolutely had to have in order to try sex with
a woman again. If it hadn't been for the medication, he would
have remained celibate the rest of his life!

Are You Ever Too Old?

We have to stop thinking of impotence as a natural occurrence
with age. It doesn't have to accompany aging. That thought probably causes more damage to people's sexual self expression than
anything else. It has a profound and insidious impact on men—
and on couples. Such thinking stops men from seeking treatment; most don't even bother to consider that there might be
something they could do to help themselves.

Both sexes will have a decrease in interest in sex as they age.
But not all people are the same. A lot of people won't think sex
is that important any more, and to them it's a bother; for others,
it is a major consideration all their lives.

A lot of men who come to me say, "I never thought this was
going to be an issue for me. I expected that as my body got older,
my interest in sex would decrease. But I realize that my body is
getting older, that I'm no longer able to get an erection, but I'm
still interested. And I realized that I could make a decision—I
could either be resigned and give it up, or I could see if there was
something I could do about it."

I think what surprises men, as they get older, is that they are
still interested in sex. They don't expect to be interested. Still,

despite the apparent contradictions, no aging man who has a problem with erections today even thought when he was young that this was eventually going to happen. I think they simply can't believe it's happening to them. They think it's an "*old man's disease.*" For it to happen in their 50s shocks them. They still feel young and think of themselves as young.

Men usually think erections are going to work forever—or are going to work whenever *they* want them to work. And suddenly they want it—and it's not working. Some men will be resigned and give it up. Some will say, let me see what else is available. However, in talking to the men who come to see me, I also get a feeling that a lot of women can either take or leave sex. Some men will say, "Well, my wife's not interested. Why should I bother?" Some will say, "Maybe she's not interested *because* I'm not performing that great anymore. Let me see what I could do about it."

If women realize this, they can find ways to counteract a man's rationalizations of disinterest in order to persuade him to seek treatment. If a woman convinces a man that she still cares about sex with him, a man is going to be a lot more interested in satisfying her by his performance. This is especially true if she lets him know that there are options, which weren't available as recently as five to 10 years ago.

That's also the challenge for doctors in this field, to actually get the word out to the patients and let them know they don't have to be resigned.

I find that many men who become very interested in sex again after a long lapse are widowers. Recently, we saw a gentleman, Mr. Y, who had colon cancer surgery and as a result could not have erections. He explained that he hadn't been very sexually active, but his wife passed away a year ago and now he's active again.

I guessed, "Well, have you a new partner?" He blushed.

Then I asked, "Have you had this new partner for a while?" He said, "Yes, I've known her for a while. It's my son's mother-in-law."

Since coming to see us, he has become active sexually using the pharmacological injection therapy.

Going On After You've Given Up

Sometimes, men who have had sexual potency problems can become very sexually active, like once a night seven days in a row. And this after they thought they'd given up sex!

At first, when people come to see me, they're prepared to be discouraged, so I see to it that they get positive feedback immediately. Some men haven't had erections in 10 or 15 years—or even more. They'll come in and with one simple injection . . . there it is. I had one patient who was almost crying, as he was telling me about the despair he felt before I did the injection. He said, "I wish I'd come sooner." He thought he had no chance because it had been so long.

"Well, don't get too excited yet because maybe nothing's going to happen," I told him. "After all, it's been over 14 years since you have had an erection." But he wanted to get one so badly, he wanted so much to believe the injections would do it, he was already nearly crying with relief.

It is interesting that many men will try having intercourse the night before they come to see me. They will tell me, "I made love last night, and you know what, it was actually a little bit better than it used to be."

I think what happens is that they have acknowledged that there is a problem, they're relieved that they're going to do something about it, and they relax a bit as they're making love. They are going to see the doctor anyway, so they feel maybe they'll just "have fun," rather than focusing on performance and worrying about whether or not it's going to work tonight.

The night before an appointment, they realize they have already started to take control of the situation. I think that's why erections sometimes get better right before they come to see me. I think it's that they've actually included the erection problem in their life, rather than trying to push it away.

Samuel Beckett says that to speak it is to bring something into existence. That means to me that to verbalize the problem is the first step one takes before getting treatment. It opens the way to action. It's a little like people who declare that they are an alcoholic. Until then, they're just heavy drinkers denying the problem. It's the same thing with erectile dysfunction (ED). To have access to treatment, a man must verbalize, must actually admit—in his mind, to us, or to his partner—that he is having problems. How can you treat a problem that doesn't exist?

Some people try to convince themselves that if you don't talk about a thing, it doesn't exist. By denying it, you continue business as usual. But when you admit to the problem, it loses some of its incapacitating energy. The upset dissipates. It becomes just something to be taken care of.

Admission is the first step on the path to treatment.

Even after acknowledging that he has a problem, and making an appointment to come to see me, a patient may still have a hard time talking about something he never told anyone before.

A man I will call Mr. J "couldn't remember" literally anything.

"Have you *ever* made love?" I asked carefully.

"Can't remember," he said.

Surely this is something a man remembers. So I asked again. Finally, he admitted: "Well, I think I did."

He thought he did. So I asked, "What do you mean you *think* you did?" (It was like trying to pin down mercury.)

"Yes, I think I did once."

Now we're getting somewhere, I thought. "So when was your last normal erection?" (This was all in line with my usual questioning in taking a man's history.)

"Can't remember," he said.

I've heard all kinds of excuses as to why erections aren't working (and probably haven't been working for a long time). "I'm not interested," "I'm too old," "I don't have the right partner." Then, too, patients insist that they can have erections and intercourse "most" of the time—but when given the test dose of medication, they get no response whatsoever, so I know they can't be getting an erection at home at all. Or often men refuse to face the reason why they came to see me in the first place.

"Can you penetrate?"

"Sure, no problem."

"Well, do you have a problem with erections?" (Supposedly the reason why they're here.)

"Yes, yes, I have a problem."

"So when was the last time you penetrated?"

"Five years ago, Doc."

It may be hard for some patients to know that on their first visit they're going to get a test injection in the office, but what has to be kept in mind is that this test serves patients best. It decreases the number of office visits, decreases the cost, is efficient, helps us reach a preliminary diagnosis quickly so that we can move on to treatment options. Once they go through that, patients see these benefits right away.

Of approximately 200–300 patients a month that I see for this problem, probably fewer than one in a hundred will refuse the initial test injection. Most often, I am the one who may refuse to do the injection because I get a sense that the problem may be totally psychological. In this situation, the patient may get a prolonged erection from the injection since the arteries are normal. So in that person, I may decline the injection even though the patient expected to have an injection and is anxious to have it.

Therefore, I have to say, "OK, we may do it—but not today. We're going to do a couple of other tests first. We're going to do a blood test, and we may also need a night test just to get a sense of what the erections are."

I find the night test is good when I suspect that there is a psychological problem, just to show the patient on a graph: Look, you had six erections that night. They were 80–100% rigid. Isn't that great? They lasted for 45 minutes. Yes, 45 minutes!

And they say, "Oh really? Really? I didn't think I had any erections while I was sleeping. Are you sure it's me?"

"Yes."

A lot of times, that's all they need.

4

A Case of Aging

Breaking the Boundaries

I encourage couples to take the first step, to seek help for faltering potency. And I urge those who may be struggling: Don't give up; don't settle for boundaries that constrict and limit your life before you've looked at *all* the options.

What has become a problem for a man can be turned into a challenge, one that can be mastered with the help of modern medicine. Potency problems do not have to be debilitating or hopeless, but rather can provide opportunities for even greater intimacy.

Understanding potency problems and choosing a treatment option can convey a kind of freedom, including freedom from the self-recrimination, shame, and guilt that faltering erections can cause. Many state-of-the-art treatment options exist today; the medical approach to erectile difficulties has changed radically in the past few years and help is as near as the closest urology specialist or erectile dysfunction center.

A Case History of Aging

People generally find it humorous that older folks want to remain sexually active. Witness cartoons, *Playboy* jibes. Grown children are often surprised—often incredulous—that their grandparents or aging parents are still interested in sex. It's as though in this culture we think that sex is only for the young, the lithe, the glamorous, and that to speak, think, dress, or act sexually later on in life is somehow in bad taste.

As we age, we seem to move into a second-class position where sex is concerned. Hollywood certainly demonstrates sexual discrimination. When was the last time you saw a romance between any couple older than their 20s—at most 30s? In fact, rarely do we see older individuals in the movies at all, much less in sexy roles, unless they are made to look as youthful, and therefore as artificial, as possible. Yet statistics show that retirees are very sexual active. This sexually forgotten and maligned group really does operate in a "closet" in order to avoid ridicule and misunderstanding.

It's easy for people who have never had problems to take a cavalier attitude about a man with erection problems, especially if the man is older but still wants to be sexually active. It's as if some people want to think that he doesn't need sex anymore, as if he shouldn't be thinking about it, as if he really doesn't have the right to be enjoying himself that way anymore. Almost as if there's something wrong with an older person still having the feelings that once were completely normal and acceptable. We tend to think he should set aside the things of youth. And this attitude still prevails. It may not be blatant, but there is an undercurrent that continues. It is helpful to be aware of this.

After undergoing a transurethral resection of the prostate (removal of the prostate through the penis without an incision),

Mr. B, a 76-year-old retired CEO, was referred to me. He had a history of coronary artery disease and peptic ulcer, enjoyed an occasional after-dinner drink—and he couldn't remember the last time he had a normal erection. He was gray-haired and looked very stylish in a navy blazer.

Mr. B and his wife came to my office together. They both looked fit. It was clear they were a team. They said they didn't want a surgical implant of artificial parts (prosthesis), but everywhere they went, they were told prosthesis, prosthesis, prosthesis. So I told them, "Let's keep that in mind, but let's put it on a back burner and see what else we can do for you."

I was moved by their obviously loving relationship. They were active people, taking walks and trips together. They liked to make love regularly. Sex was a part of their lives; it was a regular routine, but it was a healthy and joyful routine even though they had had to work out accommodations because of his faltering potency. At the same time, they kept searching for solutions, unwilling to settle for complacency, for less than a full enjoyment of life together.

Because they were older, they had encountered physicians who assumed that they didn't need what they had needed all their lives. The first doctor they had seen simply told them to forget about sex. "You've had your fun; you're over the hill. You still have orgasm, right?" He looked at Mr. B, who said, "Yes, no problem with that." So the doctor said, "Well, what's the problem then?" The wife was outraged that he totally ignored her and her needs and wishes, assuming it was her husband's dilemma alone, and not *their* problem.

Mr. and Mrs. B were grateful when I took their problem seriously even though they were not youngsters anymore. They were delighted at the possibility of continuing their original sexual relationship, especially after being told so often that they would have to accept that loss.

On the first diagnostic injection of papaverine and phentolamine, Mr. B didn't get a very good erection. So I made a special preparation for him. He was the first patient we put on a mixture of papaverine, phentolamine, and prostaglandin E_1 (Px3, we call it), which gave him an erection of 50–60%, enough to achieve penetration in intercourse.

I saw him about five months after he had been trained in self-injection. He was happy with the medication, bubbly when he talked about it. His wife also was very pleased. They had regained a powerful and important aspect of their relationship that they thought they had lost.

5

How an Erection Happens

The latest thinking on how the penis produces an erection is that there is increased inflow of blood and decreased outflow. However, it is not as simple as this.

In the first stage, an erection begins with physical stimulation. Two nerve pathways are activated once the penis is stimulated by touch. The first excites the sacral spinal cord where it activates a reflex erection. The second transmits through the sacral spinal cord to the brain to stimulate nerves there that, in turn, provoke an erection.

This is why someone with spinal cord injury who has no connection between the sacral spine and the brain can have a reflex erection, since the reflex arc—or loop—is present at the level of the pelvic area. Thus, there is an erection with no connection to the brain.

Sexually powerful psychogenic stimuli such as erotic thoughts, smells, visual stimulation, memory, and fantasies also stimulate whatever physical reflex occurs. That is why people with psychogenic problems (and remember it used to be thought that *all* erection problems were psychological) aren't able to have erections, because the psychological blocks are so powerful they can actually smother the sacral reflexes.

Men who have decreasing strength of erections (from physical causes) can benefit from being emotionally and psychologically fit because that will improve their erections. For example, if a man is under stress or if his privacy isn't secure, it's probably not a good time to make love. The better he learns to relax and be playful, the better chance he has to get a good erection.

After initial arousal, when sex is begun—or at least thought of—and mediated by the nerves connecting the brain to the penis, the sponge-like tissue inside the penis relaxes. In the flaccid (soft) state, little cavities which store blood are kept squeezed by surrounding muscle tissue. When stimulated, a substance called nitric oxide is released by the lining of these little blood cavities, by the lining of the blood vessels that feed blood into these cavities, and also by the nerve endings of the nerves which control erections. Nitric oxide serves as a potent activator of muscle relaxation. As the muscle tissue relaxes, inflow of blood into the penis increases to the expanded cavities, producing an increase in girth and length of the penis. This full relaxation results in blockage of veins that would drain blood *out* of the penis. Without full relaxation, there is a continuous leakage of blood out of the penis through these veins that are only partially blocked.

Interestingly, the highest blood flow occurs with the penis still soft but getting harder. Once the penis is very hard, there is almost no blood flow into the penis because the penis is already filled with the blood that is trapped. Thus, when a man has an erection, his blood flow can actually be lower for that short period than during the flaccid, non-erect state.

As the penis becomes totally expanded, the pressure grows very high until it reaches what we call "mean systolic pressure," which is sort of an average between the diastolic and the systolic pressure—usually about 80 and 90 mm of mercury. A man's normal mean blood pressure ranges between 120 and 100 mm of mercury. Of course, the pressure in the penis can't go higher than the blood pressure because then the blood would be flowing the other way—from the penis up to the heart instead of vice versa. Pressure generated in the penis is limited by how high a blood pressure can be generated by the heart.

In addition, if you put a little tension on an erect penis (by thrusting or slightly bending the penis during intercourse), the pressure inside can go as high as 200 mm of mercury, which is way above the pressure in the arteries of the human body. That is the pressure that occurs with thrusting during intercourse. That is what is called the rigid phase of erection.

Also, pressure goes up right before orgasm because the part of the penis that is attached to the bone has muscle around it and these muscles are squeezed so that the erection gets even harder. The head of the penis also becomes engorged.

There is evidence from penile biopsies that because of chronic lack of blood found in patients with atherosclerotic vascular disease, the muscles inside the penis are damaged and are not able to dilate. These studies show that the cells of these muscle fibers are deficient in many of the organs that are found in normal muscle cells.

A man with a low male hormone level may not have as good an erection as one with a high hormone level, since tissues react to hormones as well.

It should be noted that anything that reduces the blood pressure reduces the blood pressure inside the penis as well. That creates some problems with potency in men on antihypertension medication. They need a high head of blood pressure to bring blood through the diseased blocked arteries. Frequently, when a man sees his erection faltering, he will either stop taking antihypertensive medications, or go back to his doctor who will switch him from one medication to another, or decide on his own to take less medication. It is important to find a way to compensate for the effects of high blood pressure medications in order to continue having erections. A man will be more likely to take his antihypertensive drugs if he isn't losing his erections. Our goal in the Erectile Dysfunction Unit is to enable men (with hypertension) to have a good erection with low or normal blood pressure.

We still don't know exactly what causes certain problems, such as penile fibrosis or scarring. These terms are similar and describe a condition where the elastic inner penile tissue becomes hardened and contracted; thus losing elasticity and ability to expand and contract. One thing we do believe now, though, is that men should be somewhat careful about the way they treat their penis during intercourse. In the erect state, any lateral tension or pressure on the penile shaft, which may occur during intercourse, will increase intra-penile pressure significantly. We have no proof yet, but many specialists believe that these high pressures in the penis right before orgasm can cause trauma to the tunica of the penis resulting in microscopic tears in the lining, particularly during vigorous intercourse. This trauma causes scar tissue formation and could contribute to Peyronie's disease, which may show up when a man reaches his 50s. I find scar tissue in the penis of a lot of men I see. Instead of being smooth, the penis becomes lumpy. Calcium deposits occur so that when erect, the penis curves instead of being straight. That is Peyronie's disease.

Mr. H came to our unit and told me about the last time he had intercourse with his wife, talking as if it were yesterday. I was shocked when he told me it had happened 20 years before. He said he'd *always* had faltering erections.

On his first date with the woman who eventually became his wife, she took all her clothes off but he couldn't perform.

Nevertheless, she reassured him and they kept dating. Eventually, they tried again. This time he successfully penetrated. But erections were always troublesome.

Mr. H's wife had died two years before he came to see us. Now he was dating and he wanted to be able to have erections again. Given his history of continuing erectile difficulties, I wasn't surprised to find that he had Peyronie's disease.

What we haven't discussed yet is the detumescence phase of an erection. With good reason. That's because we still don't know why or how a man loses his erection after orgasm. When sex is initiated, you have fluids going in, fluids going out of the penis. Suddenly, the fluids going out are decreased compared to the fluids going in, and an erection results. Then, as detumescence occurs, the opposite takes place; but we don't know how.

6

The Causes of
Erection Problems

One study looking at patients who visited a general medical clinic, published in the Journal of the American Medical Association in 1983, revealed up to 34% of all men were impotent. Less than half—only 47%—of these impotent men chose to be examined for their problem. This study also found that the mean age of the impotent patients was 59.4 years.

Another article in the New England Journal of Medicine in 1978 found that up to 40% of men who were happily married, in stable relationships, reported either erectile or ejaculatory problems. That leads us to the following conclusion.

If we were to consider all men in the United States right now and look at how many of them fall within the potency risk categories, we can accurately estimate that at least 20 million men in this country alone probably have problems with erections. (This is based on the percentage of men who complain of erectile dysfunction on routine history taking during an office visit at a general medical clinic.) Because there is a nationwide problem with cholesterol, coronary/vascular disease, hardening of the arteries, high blood pressure, and the fact that the population is rapidly aging, along with the fact that prostate cancer is diagnosed at a younger age and more men are having radical prostate surgery, it becomes logical to expect that potency problems are on the increase.

It's important to understand that potency, for a man, is like having two hands and ten fingers. You grow up, your fingers are there, they're part of you, just as erections are a part of a man. At the same time, there are pressures from society in terms of performing sexually, having erections, being able to have more than one erection a day, and so on. So when suddenly this capacity, this expression and symbol of manhood, vanishes or gives signs of unpredictability, this is a catastrophe for men.

Following are some of the causes:

Blockage of the Arteries

We Americans overeat—and have way too much fat in our diets. As we have noted, a high-fat, high-cholesterol diet can eventually lead a man to erectile problems. Just as smoking and a consistently high-fat diet can harm circulation elsewhere in the body, so, too, they can damage the penile arteries. Any blockage of the arteries can ultimately lead to erection difficulties, whether partial or total, because of poor circulation at the level of the penis due to hardening of the arteries and cholesterol deposits which obstruct blood flow.

Mr. E was one such case. In his mid-50s, he had no medical problems and took no medications. He was in a new relationship and happy with it. He had an interesting presentation in that his problems occurred only at night, not in the morning. The initial screening injection test showed slight abnormality, so we gave him a nighttime study sleep test to rule out a psychological problem. Since that was also abnormal, we knew that Mr. E had mild arteriogenic dysfunction, which is perhaps the most frequent diagnosis of all. This condition cannot be cured, but erections may be improved with the use of penile injections.

Drugs

Drugs taken for medical reasons can interfere with erections. Diabetics using insulin are prone to potency difficulties; at least 50% will have problems with erections during their first year of using the drug. Diabetics on insulin might also experience retrograde ejaculation (ejaculation back or rearward into the bladder) as opposed to antegrade (normal) ejaculation. Actually, it is not the insulin that causes erection problems, but the fact that insulin is needed is an indication that metabolically accelerated atherosclerosis (plaque formation in the lumen of arteries) is present.

Any medication or drug can also affect the ability to sustain an erection. For example, cocaine narrows the arteries and can bring about angina. So people who use cocaine often use a vasodilator such as nitroglycerin or nitropace to counteract the cocaine-induced angina.

Nitroglycerin lowers the blood pressure, so the side effect of its use is that there isn't enough blood pressure to cause the penis to fill, and this causes impotence.

Any medication that lowers blood pressure, including antihypertensives or diuretics, can also cause erection problems by decreasing the pressure of blood flow into the narrowed artery. Therefore, it logically follows that it is not the medication which is the cause of the erectile dysfunction, but the underlying partial arterial obstruction.

Smoking

Statistically, around the 30 "pack year" mark, that is, when the number of packs smoked per day times the number of years smoked adds up to this figure (30), coronary artery disease and lung cancer start to appear. Researchers have discovered that cigarette smoking may be one cause of narrowing of the penile arteries, which can cause impotence. In studies, men who smoked a pack a day for five years were 15% more likely to develop blockage of the penile arteries than those who did not smoke. Smoking a pack a day for 20 years increases this percentage to 72%.

Alcohol

A man drinking alcohol may find that when he gets into bed, nothing happens. That's because alcohol binges wipe out libido, or the desire for intercourse. The body can still function, but the interest is gone. As soon as the drinking stops, erections return, unless liver damage resulting from long-term, heavy drinking is present. Over a long period (years), alcohol harms the liver. That organ stops breaking down the female hormone estrogen, a natural breakdown product of testosterone, the male hormone; then, men start having problems with erections (due to the elevation of the female hormone in the blood circulation). Still, it is rare to see that because someone with that kind of drinking problem is usually not interested in erections anymore and has much more serious health problems at that point.

Peyronie's Disease

This fibrosis or scarring of the inner spongy tissue of the penis can cause erection problems because it destroys the elasticity necessary for the penis to expand. It is not yet known why certain people develop this disease. Often, the first manifestation of this disease is an abnormal curvature of the erect penis. Erectile dysfunction can also be the first symptom of Peyronie's disease preceding pain or penile deformity.

Surgery

Prostate cancer is being discovered earlier today and treated in the years when a man is sexually vigorous, perhaps still fathering children. Men who undergo radical surgery in the pelvic area for rectum, bladder, prostate, or colon problems can sustain damage to nerves and arteries that are necessary for erections. Whether prostate surgery is "open," that is, through the abdomen, or "closed," through the penis, it can still cause erectile problems. (Historically, it was felt that only open surgery caused such problems, but it turns out that this is not the case.) Radiation therapy to the pelvic area, prostate, or bladder can also cause scarring and lead to problems with erections.

Aging

This country's population is aging and potency naturally flags with advancing years. At the same time, we see a lot of men and women who want to stay sexually active despite aging. So that is the dilemma millions of men are facing today.

The aging process alone does diminish erectile ability. Also, as men get older, many encounter the need for treatment of prostate or bladder conditions, and these treatments, too, can lead to erection difficulties. Nevertheless, men are able to have erections well into their 80s.

Today, men in their 70s and 80s continue to work, many remarry, often marrying a woman who is sexually vigorous. A new romance generally makes a man very aware and demanding of his sexual prowess. This change in negative attitudes about aging is creating a demand for better potency treatment options, such as penile injections.

Injuries

Any injury to the spinal cord, be it from a gunshot wound, knife, or any sort of trauma, can result in erectile failure, as spinal-cord trauma can damage the nerves necessary for a good erection. Those with spinal-cord injuries number about 100,000 in this country, and their number increases by at least 8,000 a year. Most of these men are young and will live for decades. New diagnostic and treatment techniques can help in these special cases, too.

Diseases

Parkinson's disease and multiple sclerosis can contribute to potency problems.

In diabetes, high glucose levels can damage some of the blood vessels that feed the nerves of the penile arteries. As these blood vessels are damaged, blood flow to the nerves dwindles, so the nerves themselves become damaged. These patients then behave just like spinal-cord-injured patients, as if the nerves had been cut. As we correct the glucose, potency returns, because the blood flow resumes and the nerves grow back again. In some cases erectile dysfunction may be the first manifestation of diabetes or multiple sclerosis.

Mr. T presented with no medical problems, no medications being taken, no history of surgery, and no drinking or smoking habits. He was in his late 40s, which is early to begin to see potency problems. His erection was only 40% of normal, although he continued to have ejaculation and orgasm.

His exam was unremarkable. A screening injection was performed, yielding a very good erection that lasted 45 minutes. However, his erections continued to be erratic. That made me suspicious, so we tested him further and it turned out that he had adult onset diabetes. After he learned to control his sugar, his erections improved, but in the meantime he was helped with the injections.

Another patient, Mr. M, came to me with a 15-year history of insulin injections for diabetes. He was 68, atherosclerotic, and depressed. He had not had an erection in that time. I wasn't too optimistic about being able to help him, but I gave him a test injection of medication to see how he might respond. With the very first dose, he got a 60% erection. At home, this pharmacological erection improved with sexual stimulation, so that he was able to penetrate.

Hormones

Patients who have had mumps or a mumps viral infection that has affected the testicles and caused them to be small with a low secretion of the male hormone testosterone will have a decreased volume of ejaculate, decreased desire for sex, and decreased sensitivity to having an orgasm. (They often complain that it takes forever to get an orgasm.) Loss of ability to maintain an erection as well as difficulty obtaining an erection may follow. Often, these men are also infertile.

Some men lose their desire to have sex because they are frustrated about erections. It's hard to know which came first: Was the libido lost first or the erection? There are clues that specialists look for in order to learn if this could be a hormonal problem.

It is important to emphasize that most men over 50 will have a hormone (testosterone) level in the 250–300 range. A lot of doctors will consider that abnormally low and will seek to increase the hormone level with testosterone injections. Testosterone injections can lead to sterility, they can increase the size of the prostate, and they can possibly promote growth of cancer cells if these are present in the prostate when the patient is started on injections. Long-term testosterone injections will also cause atrophy, or wasting, of the testicles. Why? Because the testicles' job is to produce testosterone. If there's a lot of testosterone around, the pituitary gland no longer sends the signal to the testicles to make testosterone. Without the signal, the testicles shrink. So, essentially, what happens is the patient becomes dependent for the rest of his life on the testosterone injections.

It is very important that young men not take testosterone, because it will temporarily suppress their production of sperm and they will be made sterile as long as they use this medication.

If, on the other hand, the blood test is normal and the injection test is normal, one may then go back and reassess the patient's psyche. Maybe psychogenic diagnosis was missed. Maybe the patient really has a psychological problem and the questions asked at the initial evaluation were not focused enough to pick that up.

Vein Problems (Ability to Trap Blood in the Penis)

Some men have good blood flow to the penis, but the blood doesn't get trapped there as it should. So, as the arteries pump in the blood, it flows right out of the penis and goes back into circulation. Because the "veins" don't trap the blood in the penis, a man loses his erections. A problem such as this can show up even as early as a man's teens or early 20s. This problem is known as venogenic, or abnormal veins leading to excessive leakage of blood. It is actually more complex than this. The inner penile tissues are no longer able to expand fully so as to compress the emissary veins and trap blood in the penis. This can occur in many conditions that affect the elastic tissue and muscle fibers in the penis (Peyronie's disease, trauma, muscle atrophy from plaque obstruction of blood flow).

Tumors

Sometimes a patient comes in complaining of impotence, and a brain tumor (pituitary adenoma) is eventually pinpointed that is very often curable. When the tumor is cleared up, the erection problem disappears.

Some men get tumors in an organ that makes the female hormone, estrogen, such as the adrenal. These are small glands located right above the kidneys on both sides. Such men experience impotency because the estrogen, which is secreted excessively by this tumor, interferes with their libido.

Radiation

In the 1950s, it was common to irradiate the face to cure acne. That can damage the thyroid gland, a side effect doctors weren't aware of at the time. These patients later on in life may well show up with erectile difficulties. When one corrects the thyroid hormone level, erections usually improve.

Nerves

It's very rare for just the nerves of the penis to be hit. Very rare. Usually there is nerve damage elsewhere as well. In other words, if the nerves to the penis are damaged, usually the patient will have other symptoms. For example, they will have voiding dysfunctions. Why? Because the same nerves that go to the penis for erections are the nerves that innervate the bladder. Therefore, the symptoms go together.

Exceptions can happen though. For example, lead poisoning can impair any nerve in the body. So if a patient reports painting his home and has been using lead paint or scraping old paint for a couple of months, we test for lead poisoning.

Another condition that can affect just certain nerves, especially in young men, is multiple sclerosis. One young man, Mr. C, came to us complaining of erectile dysfunction. His only other symptom was that at night, when he got tired, his vision started to blur just a little.

We did all the tests on him. He responded beautifully to the injection, and his hormone levels were normal. Psychologically, he was very stable and his history gave no indication of a mental or emotional problem. We knew it wasn't the hormones, it wasn't the arteries, and it wasn't the veins. So that left the nerves.

We sent Mr. C for evaluation of a possible spine compression from a disk problem. That turned out largely to be normal, except for one disk that was slightly pushing on the spinal cord. Because of that, the patient was referred to a neurologist to see if that disk could cause his erectile problem. It was the neurologist who, with other tests, found multiple sclerosis.

Multiple sclerosis patients sometimes experience mood swings: They are very happy, then they are very sad. It's part of the disease. One man, Mr. J, whom we saw with MS was wheelchair-bound. After he started injections, he developed priapism. He had given himself three consecutive injections because he didn't think the medication was working. As a result, he developed a very hard and large continuing erection (priapism), but he didn't come in for that even when it became painful. Instead, on one of his high moods, he had gone on a rip-roaring fling. He came back to see us only because he had developed a case of gonorrhea.

Often, what seems to be a nerve damage is another problem altogether. We frequently see patients who think theirs must be a nerve problem because they had sciatic pain in their back. A 46-year-old man, Mr. Y, developed a pinched sciatic nerve and had been seeing a chiropractor regularly for that. Then, he was found to have high blood sugar on a routine lab test, was diagnosed with diabetes, and was treated with dieting. A few years later he started on oral diabetic medications to control his blood sugar. With his diabetes under control, he recovered full erectile function. However, after taking the medication for a year, he again noticed problems with erections, so he came to see us. He described his erection as 75% of normal, so he should still have been functional. However, he couldn't penetrate. In order to become rigid enough, excessive stimulation had to be administered, then he had to rush through intercourse in order to maintain his erection. If he took his time, he lost the erection.

Still, he walked a very tight rope between ejaculation and losing the erection, because with the excessive stimulation he was very excited by the time he penetrated.

By the time Mr. Y came to me, he was ready to explode. Before this problem, he told me, all he had to do was think about sex and he got an erection. He thought his problem must have to do with his nerves because of that sciatic back pain, but it was due to the diabetes. Diabetes caused accelerated development of atherosclerosis with decreased blood flow to the penis. With painless injections he was able to obtain a fully rigid erection for 45 minutes. He took his time with intercourse and reported no reoccurrence of premature ejaculation.

Another man also thought his problems with erections were due to his sciatic nerve. He was dubious when, after testing, I told him the problem was arterial. He wasn't aware that diabetes could undercut his erections. However, he accepted the diagnosis quickly enough and turned optimistic when he saw, with injections, he was able at once to resume sexual activity with firmer erections.

Warning Signals

Slow erection, erection that depends on position (e.g., standing), erection that takes a lot of stimulation to get started, premature detumescence before orgasm, orgasm with a soft penis, all these are warning signs that the erection may steadily get worse. It's important to intervene early, because we feel it's possible to at least stop the deterioration and stabilize the problem.

The varying causes of impotence underscore the importance of providing an examining specialist with a thorough history. Pinpointing the source of the problem is essential to proper treatment. Frequently, the real cause masquerades under other seemingly unrelated symptoms. Sometimes, physical symptoms have little or nothing to do with the root of the erectile failure. That is why, too, although we include a self quiz at the end of this book, to get a true diagnosis it is important to visit a urologist who specializes in the field of erectile dysfunction.

7

The Drugs: Background

While performing penile bypass procedure in 1977, a surgeon injected papaverine in the penile arteries to cause dilation of the lumen and facilitate suturing of blood vessels. This produced a full erection of two hours' duration in this *impotent patient.* In addition, lab testing had revealed that other medications such as phentolamine (Regitine) were found to induce erections in cats when given intravenously. However, it wasn't until 1982 that Dr. Ronald Virag, a French surgeon, documented that the pressure inside the penis increased with an injection of papaverine. In 1983, a professor of physiology at the Institute of Psychiatry in London, Dr. G. S. Brindley, reported that 11 impotent men were able to have intercourse following injections. What was remarkable was that he was able to produce erections in men with *physical* problems.

He presented these findings at a major urological meeting in 1983. To make his point at the end of his talk, he stated that before starting his speech, he had injected himself to show that the erection could be induced—no matter where or how stressful the surroundings. Then he proceeded to lower his pants to let all the urologists in the room see that, indeed, he had an erection. Members of the audience even came up on stage to make sure that this wasn't a prosthesis.

It sounds theatrical, but it was done in the context of a medical meeting with only physicians present.

Several other investigators took the idea and experimented to see if they could actually use this for all kinds of physical problems. In one instance, Dr. J. Wyndaele started using the medication for spinal-cord injured males. In the U.S., in the mid-1980s, Dr. Adrian Zorgniotti at the N.Y.U. School of Medicine also took up the practice, using it on 62 men suffering from mostly vascular causes of impotence—with diabetes or atherosclerosis. Fifty-nine of these impotent men were able to achieve penetration with this treatment (Journal of Urology, 1985). Suddenly we discovered the possibility of a medically induced erection. In the late 1980s, this was one of the most discussed topics in the urological community.

Since then, there has been rapid, widespread acceptance of medically induced erections, with patient demand and preference playing a major role in promoting this treatment option.

The advent of these medications meant that a man could look at potency problems and say, "Some of the time I have a good erection, and some of the time the erection is not that great. Therefore, I'm really not impotent. I just have difficulties at times." The medications took away the heavy connotation of having erection problems. All of these drugs are approved by the FDA for use in the human body. None of the drugs are approved by the FDA for penile injections, so this is a non-dictated, non-approved use of these medications. The fact that these medications are approved by the FDA for human use allows the physician in the absence of other similar alternatives to treat with these medications even though this represents an off-label use. This is not an uncommon practice in a university setting such as ours where clinical trials are often undertaken. Currently, clinical trials are ongoing in our unit to document the efficacy and safety of these drugs in order to satisfy FDA guidelines.

The Drugs Used

Experiments with over 40 different types of medications yielded three that are most effective for patient use. Initially, papaverine hydrochloride was the one most often used. Papaverine dilates the arteries by working on the muscle cells in the arterial walls. With relaxation of the muscle wall, dilation of the artery occurs, resulting in increased blood flow into the penis. Also, blood flow out of the penis, carried by the veins, is reduced after papaverine injection, so this means that the blood is trapped there and the erection is maintained.

Papaverine has been used for over 20 years for dilation of arteries in the heart, as well as for Alzheimer's disease and multiple sclerosis. Vascular surgeons have also long used papaverine. Radiologists use it during radiological procedures involving the arteries.

Phentolamine (Regitine) replaced phenoxybenzamine because it is shorter acting, whereas phenoxybenzamine stays in the system much longer. Also, phenoxybenzamine has been implicated in producing cancer in rats, so it is not used much. Phentolamine blocks the nerves signalling arterial muscle wall contraction. Thus, when these nerves are blocked, the muscle cells in the arterial wall relax and the artery dilates. This action complements the action of papaverine. For this reason, the drugs are often used together.

The third medication used is prostaglandin E_1 (PGE_1). This is a chemical that occurs naturally in the human body. It was discovered about 30 years ago that it is a potent vasodilator. It is used in premature babies to keep their heart channels open. It also relaxes the muscle cells of the arteries of the penis, thus resulting in an erection. PGE_1 has been used only for the past three to four years to produce erections. Now it is the drug of choice for drug-induced erections.

The cost for self-injecting is variable, depending on where the medication is obtained. When a treatment unit purchases large quantities of PGE_1, the medication can be divided, mixed, and redistributed to a number of patients at lower cost.

The cost runs anywhere from $5 to $10 per injection, depending on which type of medication is used. The most costly medication is phentolamine, the second most costly is prostaglandin E1, and the cheapest is papaverine. Papaverine bottles can be obtained for under $10 for a bottle of 300 mg, which could provide as many as 20–30 injections, depending on the dose used and whether it is mixed with another medication.

The approximate cost of a two-month supply of papaverine and phentolamine with syringes generally runs in our institution around $190. PGE_1 comes in 10, 20, 30, and 40 micrograms (mcg) per cc concentration. The usual dose is 8 mcg and it comes in bottles of 10 cc, which is enough for ten doses. The cost of PGE_1 runs about $44 for a 10-cc bottle at 10 mcg/cc concentration, and this includes both syringes and needles.

We mostly use prostaglandin E_1 because studies have shown it to be safer, and it is a more specific vasodilator than papaverine, which is nonspecific. PGE_1 binds reversibly, meaning that the molecules of PGE_1 can come off the receptor that causes vasodilation, whereas papaverine is irreversibly bound so the cells need to metabolize the receptor to get rid of the papaverine. That means it takes longer to bring down the erection. The potential side effects such as penile scarring, formation of nodules, fibrosis, and prolonged erections are much smaller or absent with

PGE_1. However, papaverine is more powerful than PGE_1 and some patients just don't get an erection with PGE_1 but get a nice erection with papaverine. So we use papaverine in that group of patients.

In addition, PGE_1 sometimes causes a temporary dull ache in the penis. We don't know whether this ache is based on the fact that the currently available PGE_1 is in alcohol, or if it is due to the saline it is mixed in, or if it is due to the molecule of PGE_1 itself. This doesn't happen in every patient.

We have used up to 100 mcg of PGE_1 in patients; with papaverine, we have gone up to 120 mg for penile injections. When patient doses get to be that high and the erection is not as good, patients are usually much happier with a penile implant and we recommend an implant in that setting.

The number of injections should not exceed 12 a month, and we recommend that injections be spaced evenly. Also, the site of injection should alternate between the right and left side of the penis so that scarring is minimized.

An erection occurs anywhere from 10 to 20 minutes following the injection. In general, PGE_1 works slightly faster than papaverine and phentolamine. A better erection is usually obtained after some foreplay. The injection may be administered before or after foreplay, and men are encouraged to experiment to see what works the best. Some men may require a 30-minute wait before getting a fully rigid erection. In general, the amount of time that it takes to obtain an erection is a correlate of the extent of arterial blockage.

Pharmacological erections generally last anywhere from 20 minutes to an hour and a half.

The papaverine and phentolamine mixture is effective for 60 days. Dr. Lloyd Allen of the University of Oklahoma College of Pharmacy studied the stability of the mixture and showed that when it is stored in a refrigerator at 40 degrees Fahrenheit, papaverine lost less than 3% of its activity and phentolamine less than 7%. PGE_1 kept refrigerated at 40 degrees Fahrenheit will last for four months.

The pharmacological treatment has been successful in producing erections in over 80% of the patients seen in our Erectile Dysfunction Unit. The erections are more than adequate to perform intercourse. The rest of the patients for whom injections are not effective are candidates for other forms of treatment.

Injections are not a treatment. They do not cure or reverse the blockage of the arteries. They simply allow the individual to obtain an erection without surgery or other means. They may not continue to work if the condition (i.e., high cholesterol, high blood pressure, etc.) continues to affect the penile arteries. Tobacco smoking can also affect erectile function to the point where the injections will not work, and we tell all patients to stop smoking.

Erections produced by injections do not interfere with the capacity to have an orgasm. Generally, men who are able to achieve orgasm without a firm erection before they come for treatment will continue to reach orgasm when having an erection by injection.

The men who are candidates for the Pharmacological Erection Program are those who can obtain an erection with injections. Contraindications to penile injections include sickle cell disease, and poor manual dexterity or poor vision.

8

Workup for Potency

The Pharmacological Erection Program at The New York Hospital–Cornell Medical Center is aimed at getting men functioning as soon as possible. The best tools for evaluating a patient suffering from erection problems are: 1) history taking, and 2) the physical examination, including the penile injection test.

History Taking

We feel that the most important part of the workup with a man who has erection problems is the history taking, sitting with the patient, asking detailed questions, and not being embarrassed to talk about the situation in detail. We ask, for example, whether or not the patient masturbates, how his erection is with masturbation, how his erection is with ejaculation. Then we talk about the last time the patient penetrated: Was penetration better in a certain position than in another? These may seem like unrelated details, but they are important. In the past, we've relied too much on invasive, complicated, expensive procedures. We have moved away from that approach, which comes as a surprise to many patients, and we actually go from history taking directly to treatment, since we know that most patients who suffer from erection problems have decreased circulation, blocked arteries, and decreased blood flow to the penis. In addition, most patients do not want surgery or a penile prosthesis. (The self quiz on pp. 143–151 covers the same questions asked in a history-taking session.)

The following is our systematic approach to getting down to where the problem is.

PAST MEDICAL HISTORY

First, we want to know about past medical history. Are there any past illnesses or medical conditions that could be risk factors for erectile dysfunction? Does the patient have a history of heart attack? If he does, we know he has evidence of blocked arteries. Could he possibly have the same problem in the penis as he does in the heart? Yes. Atherosclerosis is a systemic disease occurring throughout the entire body. It affects the coronaries, the carotid arteries to the brain, the femoral arteries to the lower extremities, and the arteries to the penis. The same assumption applies if the patient has history of a stroke. Or if a patient has hypertension, which could indicate hardening of the arteries. All these are risk factors.

We ask if the patient had any previous surgery, particularly paying attention to any type of major pelvic surgery: Radical prostatectomy can cause impotence. Any radical surgery for colon cancer that involves major pelvic surgery can cause impotence. Nerves and arteries can be severed during surgery, and this could be the cause of impotence.

Radiation therapy for colon or prostate cancer is associated with problems with erections. It accelerates atherosclerosis and produces a reaction in the walls of the arteries, in that the arteries become thickened and the lumen becomes obstructed.

Finally, medications play a role. Inderal, beta blockers, as well as alpha methyl dopa, reserpine, and some antihistamines have been associated with erection problems. We have a list of medications that can worsen erections. In general, though, medications adversely affect or take away an erection *only* if there is an underlying problem. If arteries are normal, these medications do not actually *cause* potency problems. However, with abnormal arteries, they may play a role. In that case, withdrawing these medications may be sufficient to provide the patient with an erection.

Sometimes, of course, we can't cancel out a patient's medications. For instance, if a patient has high blood pressure, we can't take his antihypertensive medication away. However, some of our treatment options allow these patients to be compliant with the medications that keep them alive, that play a key role in their health, and at the same time make it possible for them to enjoy sex.

Smoking is particularly important because we know coronary artery disease and hardening of the arteries are associated with tobacco smoking. A lot of our patients are tobacco smokers. We recommend that they stop so that they don't contribute to worsening the disease.

Drinking, especially if the patient complains of erectile failure during binges, obviously could be the cause of erection problems. We see that particularly in young males between 16 and 20. They tend to drink 10 or more beers on a Saturday night, then around 1:00 in the morning, they get worked up and try to have sex.

SOCIAL HISTORY

We go into the status of the patient: Is he married, single, divorced? Is this a second marriage? What is the quality of his relationship with his partner? What is his sexual preference? I had a patient, Mr. B, who had great erections with men, but could not get an erection with women. He wasn't a declared homosexual and he wanted to have the option of being with both men and women. Then, he met a woman, fell madly in love with her, and for 20 years, they had a great marriage. He was faithful, never had intercourse with any other woman—or man—during that time. When his wife died of breast cancer, he was devastated. A week after she died, he went out meeting men. His homosexual encounters were strictly for sex and he had great erections. But now the plot thickens, as it seems prone to do. He met not one but two ladies, spent time with them, and with both of them—nothing, nothing, nothing. He feels that ladies are attracted to him, he has a lot of lady friends, but his erections don't work with them. Yet he really wants to have sex with a woman. He's a bit confused at this stage.

That history is important information because it tells me there's nothing *physiologically* wrong with his erections.

It is also important for me to know if the relationship has some friction. Sometimes I have to delve deeper. Perhaps the spouse is not interested in sex anymore. Her husband doesn't get an erection, he gets frustrated, he thinks that he doesn't get an erection because she's not stroking and touching him and being responsive, and he puts the blame on her. She gets angry and is turned off even more by sex, so she says, "I'm not interested." These matters can be more complex than sometimes is apparent at first. And the whole problem may be that he doesn't have good erections and that's why she's not interested. Maybe she would be interested if he could perform.

We want to know whether the patient's partner wants to have the problem corrected. Some partners are happy with the way things are. If that's the case, we support the patient even more because he's not going to have the support of his partner.

These are some of the things we look for in the history taking. We also ask if the patient has consulted a psychiatrist in the past, if he is in a crisis right now. When a man is having difficulties with his partner, it may not be the best time to evaluate his erection because there are overlying psychological factors. We may want to wait a bit, reassure the patient, and check him later when things calm down.

LIBIDO

Then we spend some time studying his libido, which is the *desire* for sex. We want to distinguish here a loss of libido that is due to psychological causes from a loss of libido from hormonal causes. Testosterone, the male hormone, is mostly responsible for libido. Men with low serum testosterone describe these symptoms: 1) decreased desire for sex; 2) inability to maintain an erection; 3) decreased volume of ejaculate; 4) decreased sensation in the penis; 5) more time needed between sex to build up an erection again; 6) decreased number of sexual fantasies. We ask questions probing these areas.

If a patient has lost his job and is somewhat depressed, his libido may go down. However, on physical exam he has healthy, large, firm testicles with normal male distribution of hair and healthy muscle bulk, and most likely the patient will have a normal testosterone level.

It should be noted that testosterone level does go down as a man ages. For a patient who is 60 to 70, testosterone level in the 300 range is absolutely normal and should not be corrected. It should be corrected only if it is less than 100.

Testosterone replacement usually works on a temporary basis on the well-selected patients who need it. Usually, replacement doesn't work on patients with simply low testosterone. It has to be *abnormally* low.

ERECTIONS

Once we have teased out some of the answers regarding libido, we follow this up with questions about erections themselves. When did the problem start, and was it acute or gradual? If it was gradual, the problem is most likely organic; if acute, the problem is probably psychological. Before the problem started, how often did the patient have intercourse? That also tells about the libido as well as the patient's interest and motivation in getting help. We want to know how often the patient attempts intercourse now. What percent of the time is he able to penetrate? Sometimes I see patients who say they can't have sex anymore. I ask how many times they tried. They tell me they tried twice.

Has the penis shape changed? If it has changed, that suggests Peyronie's disease. Patients with Peyronie's disease have difficulty maintaining an erection. Usually, Peyronie's disease alters the veno-occlusive mechanism of the penis (the ability of the penis to trap blood); as a result, patients experience softening of the erection.

Is the patient able to have a partial erection? If yes, the problem is most likely organic. If not, it is most likely a psychological problem. If there is severe blockage of the vessels, the patient will have nothing. Usually, that patient will also have other risk factors or be a tobacco smoker. If I see a young male who tells me he has *no* erections whatsoever, I suspect that his problem is psychological.

Does the patient have difficulty maintaining the erection? Again, that is most likely physical rather than psychological etiology.

Does the patient ejaculate with a soft penis? A very good question, but very seldom asked of patients because it is embarrassing to ask about ejaculation. Most patients with erectile dysfunction answer yes. Why? Because it is very rare for a man with normal vasculature to the penis to ejaculate with a soft penis. It can happen, but it's very rare. If a patient ejaculates with a soft penis consistently, we know the problem will turn out to be physical.

Then we ask the patient about the quality of his erection: Is it totally limp? Is it a full penis, but is there no hardness and no penetration? Is it firm enough for occasional penetration, but with no maintaining ability? Is it hard enough for sufficient penetration all the time, but does it go down before orgasm? Or is it able to penetrate easily and maintain to orgasm?

Then we want to know how the erection is when he's not with a partner, when he doesn't have to perform. Is it the same or is it better? If better, the problem is psychological. If it is the same or worse, the problem could be physical.

Does he get erections at night while sleeping? Are erections present in the morning? If they are, it suggests only that the patient gets night erections. It doesn't mean that the patient can have sexual erections, but it does provide us with some information. If a patient is young, but cannot get satisfactory erections with a partner, for example, but tells us that he has great morning erections, we know he has a psychological problem. On the other hand, if an older patient says he has morning erections, his dysfunction could still have a physical cause. Why? Because older men will get morning erections even if they have blocked arteries to the penis, even if they have an abnormality of blood flow to the penis. Still, a lot of older men are diagnosed as having psychogenic erectile dysfunction (ED) based on the fact that they told someone that they had morning erections.

So we move on with our questions. How do these morning erections compare with their sexually induced erections? Does their ability to have erections vary with different partners? If a man is bisexual, that may happen.

Is the patient able to have climax or orgasm? Does semen

come out? If the volume of semen is down, this is possibly hormonal. Has the sensitivity of the penis changed? With this, we're looking for neurological causes such as lead poisoning, multiple sclerosis, diabetes.

In sum, this is basically what we want to know from the patients when they first come to see us.

The Physical Exam

At this Erectile Dysfunction Unit, an initial workup also consists of a physical examination, blood drawing, and a test dose of injection in the penis. Rarely do we find any gross physical abnormalities. Most of the time, the man will have normal testicles, a normal penis, a normal abdomen, palpable pulses in both extremities, and a normal rectal exam.

The Combined Injection and Stimulation Test

After the physical exam, a man is injected in the penis with a standard dose of medication, either papaverine/phentolamine or prostaglandin E_1. This test is actually less expensive and more accurate than other more complicated studies.

We start with this test because it is aimed specifically at arterial disease, since we know that 90% of all the patients who come to see us have problems with blood flow. In addition, we are a society of meat and egg eaters, so we often have high cholesterol. The group of men who used to eat two eggs every morning is now becoming older, and this type of diet produces this problem.

Another factor is that our population is aging, and we know

that people generally develop hardening of the arteries as they get older.

If patients come in with a medical problem such as diabetes or high blood pressure, we can still test them with injection of these medications. That is the other point that makes this medication a powerful tool: There is scarcely a person you cannot safely inject. Perhaps the only person you can't inject is a patient with a penile implant. But people on blood thinners, such as Persantine or Coumadin; people with heart problems or high blood pressure; diabetics or transplant patients—all can be injected. In fact, we have cardiac patients and renal transplant patients, among others.

The reason we can inject almost anyone is that the drugs are extremely mild and the volume used is insignificant compared to the total blood volume in the body. Plus, the medication is active only locally. It is better than taking a pill, because it doesn't act on your brain cells, it doesn't act on your heart cells, it just acts on the penis. By the time it gets out into the blood stream, it is so diluted it has no general effect.

We do know that when you give a man a penile injection of a medication that dilates arteries, an erection will result. This erection can be enhanced by stimulation of the nerves of the penis, or by visual erotic stimulation, or by manual stimulation. These facts are used in evaluating a patient with erection problems.

Use of medications to evaluate erections is a breakthrough in this field. Before the effects of these drugs on erections were discovered, we had a tremendous number of tests, such as nocturnal penile tumescence studies, nerve conduction studies, penile blood pressure tests, arteriography to look at the arteries, etc. There were so many, yet we could rarely make a definite diagnosis.

The great advantage of penile injections is that this constitutes a dynamic study. In other words, we are actually *looking* at the patient as the patient is having an erection. No other test gives us that. We can actually *see* the problem in progress and calculate what is the maximum dose of medication that this patient can tolerate in order to get a short-term erection.

If a patient complains of penile curvature, we actually get to see the curvature, rather than seeing a Polaroid picture or evaluating the penis through electrical charting while the patient is asleep (nocturnal study).

Initially, of course, on their first visit most men are concerned about having a needle stuck into their penis. Actually, it's a very small needle, much smaller than the one diabetics use to inject themselves, and this makes the sticking painless. It's the smallest sterile needle made, and men usually tell me they "didn't feel a thing." Fewer than 10% of my patients are concerned about the needle after their first encounter with injections.

The patient stands to receive the injection and remains standing (to take advantage of the boost of gravity). Meanwhile, the patient reads sexually stimulating magazines or watches a sexy video to make the test truer. He is left alone and asked to masturbate to maximize the effect of the injection. This also tells us if the patient is at risk of obtaining a prolonged erection when he'll be doing this at home on his own. So, masturbating in the office in the standing position with an injection is critical because it determines the maximum effect that the medication can have on a patient. His erection is examined at five and 15 minutes.

At first, men are embarrassed about getting this test and about getting an erection in the office. It is difficult for them, especially when they are asked to masturbate after the injection. However, I feel that if I have a relaxed attitude they are going to be relaxed. Also, I tell them *why* I am asking them to do this. Masturbation is the most powerful stimulation to the penis known to man—more powerful than the vagina, more powerful than oral sex. That is why we use it in the office. Once patients understand the reasoning behind this, they actually can't wait until I leave the room, because they want to participate, they want to see for themselves.

"Yes, I want to see if I get harder with the injection and stimulation, because I have been having some buckling in the erection." That's the kind of thing a man will tell me.

So I'm matter-of-fact about the testing, and even if a man is embarrassed at first, he gathers support from my stance. Men relax and see that it is not so hard as they thought. They then can talk about their erections; after all, it's just a medical problem, nothing else. It's as if they were talking about their high blood pressure. Nothing embarrassing about that.

If the erection obtained in the office is good enough for penetration and the erection subsides spontaneously, it suggests that this is a problem with blood circulation in the penis. It also tells us that the patient can use this method to assist intercourse at home.

Then the patient evaluates his own erection.

We also assess the erection and grade it from zero to 5 (5 being a rigid erection, zero being no response whatsoever). We grade the erection according to a standardized method. We look for fullness, fullness with buckling, fully rigid, and so on. If a partial erection is noted at 15 minutes following the injection, and if manual/genital stimulation (masturbation) results in a rigid erection of 20 minutes or more, what this indicates to us is that: a) the patient's reflexes are working, since the nerves of the skin improved the erection; b) the fact that the erection maintains itself indicates that the veins are doing their job in trapping blood in the penis; and c) there is no psychological inhibition, since the patient has actually masturbated and had a full erection.

The test can also indicate that this patient does not have any major psychological hangups. However, even if he does, it is still possible that he might get an erection with the medication. Or he might have no psychological hangups and still not get a full erection. So the injection is not entirely foolproof, but we balance out this test with the history taking, which is why that part is crucial.

If the erection is maintained during the test, this indicates that the patient may or may not have arterial insufficiency. Therefore, it doesn't distinguish if there is an arterial problem. It just *rules out other causes.* That is why the medication is so useful, because it can rule out a lot of other possible problems such as hormones or the nerves.

If the patient gets a tremendous erection at five minutes, that indicates that the arteries and penile muscle tissue are healthy. We then follow through with a blood test to check the hormones. If there are any neurological abnormalities, the patient will be referred to a neurologist to make sure that he doesn't have a nerve injury, multiple sclerosis, or some other disease that affects nerves.

If the erection response is adequate, we know that injections could be the treatment of choice. With the injection, not only do we see if an erection can be produced, we see how hard it gets, how long it stays up, if it can be used for intercourse.

In addition, an injection given on the first visit for diagnostic purposes gives the patient a sense of how painless it is. He also sees dramatically how effective the medication can be as he sees himself getting a rock-hard erection. Sometimes, that's the only therapy a man needs, to see for himself that he's "normal." Men leave our offices feeling upbeat and in a happy state of mind. Many have told me they feel almost "high," knowing that, "Wow, I got an erection today like I haven't had for the last 15 years. And you know what? It was really easy and simple. And you know what? I can't wait to start this and to be able to function again and be happy."

We don't necessarily need to know the diagnosis in order to treat. Very often we don't know what the problem is, yet we give penile injections. Why? Because all other treatment alternatives are not acceptable to the patient. Therefore, I believe that any additional diagnostic procedures will not alter the treatment and, therefore, don't serve the patients.

9

Further Testing and Followups

I spend a lot of time explaining to my secretaries, "You may actually be the first person outside of this man's wife or maybe not even his wife, you may be the first person in the world whom that man calling for an appointment is letting know that he has a problem with erections. Men wish they didn't have to go through this."

The first visit, most men are uptight. But when they come back a second time, they're never embarrassed. The second time, they say hello to everybody. It's a whole new ball game.

Second Visit

From the response to the injection test on the first visit, we gain a good sense of what the patient diagnosis is. On this second visit, we start to talk about options because this determines where the patient will go from here.

It is a little tricky at this point to get an idea of how far the patient is willing to go. If a patient is not interested in surgery, or not interested in anything invasive, then his options are: 1) to do nothing, 2) use penile injections, 3) use a vacuum device. We don't need to do an extensive workup at that point. Previously, people were treated as if they were on an assembly line; everybody was getting the same workup. Now it's individualized according to:

a. the patient's age
b. his motivation
c. what he wants and expects
d. other medical conditions

The patient is always given a diagnosis, and the diagnosis is documented in the chart before we proceed with treatment.

Erectile dysfunction—or impotence—is *not* a diagnosis. *It is a symptom.* It is like fever. Fever is not a diagnosis. It is a symptom, for example, of an abscess, an autoimmune disease, or just the flu. There are a limited amount of signals the body can send to let us know that we have a problem, and a lot of diseases use the same signal. So, again, we have to find the diagnosis. A diagnosis would be: arterial disease, venoocclusive dysfunction, nerve damage, hormonal dysfunction, or psychological dysfunction. All of these are diagnostic labels of the problem.

What makes a person a specialist is the ability to make fine distinctions, where someone else cannot. Thus, a general urologist (depending on his/her training) may not be able to make those distinctions that make all the difference in the diagnosis of erectile dysfunction. And treatment rests on a correct diagnosis, as well as on the patient's preferences.

Further Testing

DOPPLER ULTRASOUND TEST (DUPLEX)

If the patient doesn't get a full erection with the initial test injection, we follow up with a repeat injection and possibly a Doppler ultrasound test.

With the pulsed Doppler study, we scan the penis in the flaccid state, then reexamine the patient after an injection. This is the most reliable test to evaluate the arteries in the penis. The Doppler measures blood flow. Ultrasound measures the dilation of the artery. Without the injection, this test is not useful.

First, we use ultrasonography to measure the *diameter* of the artery in the resting state. After the injection, we again measure the artery and note the difference in diameter. That gives us an idea as to whether or not the artery is healthy and dilates as it should with stimulation. If the arteries are normal, we expect them to dilate. The Pulsed Doppler is utilized to look at the increase in *blood flow*. Once the artery is dilated, we apply the Doppler under ultrasound guidance. So we are not Dopplering any other arteries in the penis. (With the old Doppler method, we would accidentally pick up the superficial arteries of the penis. This Doppler is specifically aimed with the ultrasound at the *central* artery in the penis.) Once we're focused on the artery, we turn on our Doppler and measure the flow.

We expect an increase in blood flow in the penis with arterial dilation. No increase in flow occurs if the larger arteries supplying blood to the penile arteries have been narrowed by plaque. If the problem is a venous leak, there will be no erection despite normal arterial dilation and normal blood flow.

We look at the wave/curve pattern, how the flow increases and decreases with each heartbeat. This is an indication of whether or not there is arterial obstruction of inflow of blood to the penis. If we see good dilation of the artery but there's *no* follow through with increased blood flow, that means there is obstruction *upstream* at the level of the major vessels.

If, on the other hand, you have no dilation and no increase in blood flow, then that indicates that the arteries of the penis itself are hardened and have atherosclerosis. We know this because we have done this test in normal men, and we know what the dilation should be and what the flow should be.

This test confirms—or rules out—the diagnosis of arterial disease.

There is no discomfort associated with the procedure. Some men develop a small bruise at the injection site which resolves within seven to 10 days. If the problem is psychological, a man will develop a full erection that can last for hours, but after an hour we aspirate blood from the penis to relieve the pressure and bring down the erection. An antidote is subsequently given to prevent further erections.

Now, if that test is normal, then it's possible that the problem may be hormonal. But we would have picked that up with blood tests, which are routinely done on a first visit.

THE SLEEP TEST

In our Unit this is no longer an initial screening test as it was postulated to be years ago. We use it as an adjunct, but it is no longer at the top of our armamentarium of diagnostic tools. The nocturnal—or sleep—study came about because doctors noted that little boys or premature male infants had erections during sleep. These erections were frequent. A child may have eight to 12 erections during sleep; as a man grows older, the frequency decreases and as few as three per night are normal. These nocturnal erections are associated with REM sleep. They are also associated with a full bladder. It seems that the local pelvic nerve pathways that are utilized to close the urinary sphincter during sleep (so that a man is not incontinent when the bladder is full) are also doing something—we don't know exactly what—to cause a nocturnal erection.

Actually, that is one of the main reasons why many men don't seek treatment. They are convinced their problem is in their head because they wake in the morning with an erection and so they assume that their sexual erection is working. They think they're not excited, or they're suppressed, or not interested, when they're with their wives, and they conclude that the problem is psychological.

A lot of men tell me, "Gee, if I just could have my morning erections to have sex, it would be great. But I don't, Doc. I get a morning erection, I go to urinate, I come back, and we try to make love, but the erection goes right away."

Or, "I'll wake up my wife at 4:00 in the morning because I have an erection, and I turn over to penetrate, and the erection gets lost. Or my wife is asleep and not willing."

However, nocturnal erections are not entirely similar to sexual erections, but are based on a different mechanism.

Psychiatrists, sex therapists, and urologists used to think that if a man could have erections while sleeping and none when awake, it therefore meant the problem was in his head, because obviously his consciousness affected his erections. A large number of men were diagnosed with psychological problems because they had nocturnal erections and no erections while awake.

Now we know that if you don't have erections at night, all it means is that you don't have them at night. It doesn't signify anything about the day period.

The nocturnal study has a limited use because we know today that men who have physical problems can have good nocturnal erections. In the beginning, these tests were poorly done.

Some tests looked only at the girth of the penis, not at how hard it became. A man with a full but limp penis would break the test-snap gauges and be categorized as having psychogenic erectile dysfunction, yet the penis was not rigid at all during sleep.

Some physicians started doing these tests in hospitals, where they monitored brain waves at the same time. The patient had something hooked up to his penis and something hooked up to his brain, in unfamiliar surroundings, with a medical student observing him to count the number of erections while he slept. How can you sleep like that? Then they gave him medications for sleep, and once they did that, they altered the basis of the test. These sleep labs became popular in the 1960s and '70s. They charged a lot, but didn't contribute significantly to the clinical management of a lot of these patients.

Finally, it became clear that rigidity as well as girth must be measured. Yet, even doing that with portable units that the patient takes into his home and sleeps with, there are drawbacks such as being uncomfortable from the machine and not sleeping well, which alters the result. But most important, we know now that each case is different.

If a patient is young and has great erections at night with a sleep test, most likely he has a psychological problem. Sometimes, after we give a young patient an injection in the penis and he doesn't get an erection, we may want to find out if he was very anxious in the office or if he has a problem at night, too. Most often, if a patient doesn't respond to an injection in the office, he will have an abnormal night study. But if he is older and has a couple of firm erections, mostly in the morning when he's about to awaken with a full bladder, then that man could still be totally impotent. He might have partial erections insufficient for penetration. We can't use that test for an older man.

The history taking serves us much better, because the older man tells us exactly what is going on. He may think it's in his head, but after he gives you a history of gradual worsening erections, ejaculation with a soft penis, great relationship with his wife, I know it's going to be physical. If a younger man with an acute problem, with no erections at all, has an erection with one woman and not the other, or no erections in the beginning of a relationship until he gets used to his partner, I know it's psychological, so we don't need the sleep test in any event.

The test itself involves two to three nights. The Rigiscan is a unit that is computerized and counts the number of erections, the rigidity of each, and the change in girth of each erection. A gauge like a rubber band fits at the base and tip of the penis. These bands are activated so that they will measure girth and, in addition, squeeze every 15–30 seconds so that they sample rigidity. A computer the size of a small book fits in a pocket that a man wears on his leg. It's not too pleasant, but it's not painful. It's just uncomfortable sleeping with two of these gauges on your penis and with a computer strapped to your leg. When the study is completed, it is returned to the doctor who unloads it into the main computer program. A printout of how many erections you had, how hard they got, and how frequently they occurred is obtained. Perhaps the greatest drawback to the sleep test is recent evidence that the results on each individual patient are not reproducible.

DYNAMIC INFUSION CAVERNOSOMETRY-CAVERNOSOGRAPHY (DICC)

DICC is a test to evaluate the extent and location of abnormal leakage of blood from the penis during an erection. In some patients, the presence of abnormal veins draining the penis explains why an erection is not obtained—or maintained. This test is designed to identify these veins.

The DICC procedure is performed in conjunction with a radiologist and usually involves x-rays. In the cavernosometry part, we can precisely measure the fluid changes within the penis during an erection. First, we measure the internal pressure of the resting penis. Then papaverine and phentolamine are injected into the base of the penis to stimulate an increase in blood flow and produce an erection. After 10–15 minutes, the pressure in the penis is remeasured. A water and salt solution (saline) is infused to artificially produce a firm "normal" erection. The rate of infusion necessary to maintain a full erection is recorded. The pressure is increased and the rate of decline after stopping the saline is also measured.

Having completed the cavernosometry part of the procedure, dilute x-ray contrast solution is infused and x-rays taken. The combination of pressure measurements and radiological evaluation helps to exclude or confirm the diagnosis of abnormal venous leakage. These special x-ray studies can pinpoint problems such as scar tissue, arterial blockage, venous leakage, and abnormal vascularity, all of which can affect an erection. Usually, these x-rays are taken only when necessary to precisely locate these abnormalities.

ANGIOGRAPHY

Angiography is never performed as a screening test in individuals with erectile dysfunction. This test is reserved for a small, selected group of patients for whom reconstructive surgery is contemplated. Studies of the arteries themselves may show some minimal alteration of the blood vessels, but will fail to give information regarding the structure of the penis itself. For that, you need a biopsy that can be evaluated by a pathologist with a microscope. Further, angiography of the penis is an extremely difficult procedure that is operator dependent, and we are still struggling with interpretation of results from this study.

This is why many of us in the field of erectile dysfunction

feel that the best study is a dynamic one, which looks at the penis both in the flaccid and erect states. Ideally, it would be great to study the blood flow of the penis in a natural situation. Since that's almost impossible to do, we use the small injection at the base of the penis to stimulate the blood flow. This may not be similar to a naturally occurring erection; however, this injection combined with duplex ultrasonography gives us an idea of how the artery dilates and how fast the blood flow increases. This, I believe, is currently the best available method of study.

10

Why Injection Therapy

Choosing an Option

When treatment options are discussed with a patient, each option is reviewed with particular attention to benefits versus risks and complications, so that everything is assessed. Depending on the diagnosis, of course, options can include doing nothing, sexual therapy, using an external vacuum tumescence device, hormone replacement, penile prosthesis implant, surgical revascularization, or pharmacological self-injections. In my opinion, the two most effective treatment options for organic erectile dysfunction are penile self-injections and penile prosthesis implantation.

Once you get a sense of what an erection feels like on penile injection medications, of how painless it is, of how quickly it can produce an erection, and of how effective and reliable the medication is, making a decision for self-injections comes easily. If you can get an erection with a doctor in a white coat examining you in a brightly lit room, think of what you could do in the bedroom where everything is more erotic and stimulating. Men understand that.

PENILE IMPLANTS

As with any surgical option, penile implants are an invasive step which is best held out as a backup option after other less invasive alternatives have been tried. There is no enhancement of residual, albeit diminished, erectile capacity. In order to create space for the implant cylinders to fit into the body of the penis itself, one unavoidably destroys the remaining capability of the penis to become erect.

Men who do not respond to penile injections at home, however, most likely have little or no residual erectile capacity. (Lack of response in the doctor's office is not as significant as lack of response to injection in the home setting.) In these cases, placement of penile prosthesis becomes an appropriate alternative, since no significant erectile tissue remains.

The first penile implants were rigid and involved placement of a rib or silicon-covered wire beneath the skin of the penis. In the early '60s, a rod was placed deep within the penis rather than superficially. These produced a constant erection. Needless to say, none of these alternatives was especially popular.

Then in the early 1970s, Dr. Brantley Scott developed the first inflatable prosthesis that mimics a natural erection. Since then, over one hundred thousand have been implanted in the United States alone. This soft elastic mechanical device, capable of expanding and contracting without losing elasticity, provides a flaccid, soft penis, and, when inflated, a rigid and long-lasting erection. Currently the most physiologically realistic prosthesis is the Ultrex-Plus (American Medical Systems). It consists of three main components: 1) cylinders, which fit deep in the center of the shaft of the penis; 2) the pump, which is placed in the scrotal sac; and 3) the reservoir, which is placed deep in the pelvis behind the abdominal muscles. The reservoir contains fluid, which when transferred into the cylinders, produces expansion in width and length

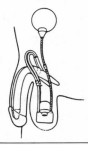

Figure 1 *Penis with prosthesis in the flaccid state. The cylinders are fitted deep in the shaft of the penis, the pump is placed inside the scrotal sac next to one of the testicles, and the fluid reservoir is placed behind the muscles deep in the abdomen.*

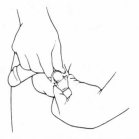

Figure 2 *By simply squeezing and releasing the pump, fluid is transferred from the reservoir to the cylinders.*

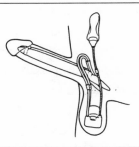

Figure 3 *The expandable cylinders are full, resulting in an erection. A release valve at the bottom keeps the fluid in the penis until intercourse is completed.*

as well as increased rigidity. The entire device can be placed through a two-inch incision in the scrotal area. Malfunction rates are low, less than 5% for the first five years, with life expectancy of a modern inflatable prosthesis ranging from eight to 15 years. (Fig. 1–Fig. 3) Courtesy of American Medical Systems, Inc., Minnetonka, Minnesota. Medical illustrations by Michael Schenk.

J.R., 62 years old, was in good health except for penile dysfunction. We determined that he suffered from arteriogenic problems and treatment options were discussed with him. He preferred self-injections and began the PEP program with us. Because he is right-handed, he favored injecting himself on the right side and this led to scarring and a curvature of the penis. (This can occur with Papaverine, but has not yet been seen with Prostaglandin E_1.) It was evident that this was not a long-term option for J.R. anymore.

J.R. and his wife, 18 years younger than he, decided that an implant would give them the best opportunity for a healthy, active sex life for the longest time. Various implants were shown and described to them; risks and possible complications were analyzed. The implant was placed.

Three weeks later at his post-op visit, J.R. was taught to inflate and deflate the device. Six weeks later, he sent a note from a long vacation he and his wife had decided to take: "We're more intimate than we have been in years—and not just physically!"

The bottom line is that all conservative options should be tried, but if these fail, the penile prosthesis remains an excellent long-term and highly satisfactory option.

Use of the Injections

If a man wishes to pursue a course of treatment in the Pharmacological Erection Program after the first visit, he returns for the "home trial visit." During this visit, the patient performs his first self-injection in my presence. If the original injection on the first visit did not yield a good erection, the mixture for the injection is changed or increased the second time around. Therefore, the second visit serves two purposes: to try another medication, if necessary, and to teach the patient how to perform self-injection. He also learns how long he can count on his medically induced erection to last, because a lot of men worry that it's going to quit on them too soon.

After the second visit, the patient is given three prefilled syringes with different doses for a home trial. He will try these on his own. These are prefilled so the patient doesn't have to worry about filling the syringe on his first home injection. After self-injecting with these syringes at home, the patient returns, reports on which one worked best, and is given a prescription for that medication. He is also taught how to fill the syringes and the informed consent is explained and signed.

We also tell patients not to expect too much the first two or three times they are injecting. We say, "You probably will have a better erection than you've been having on your own, but it may not be that much better." We tell them, "This is a test. You're not in the treatment phase yet, so don't expect anything. You're going to be nervous about injecting yourself, and if you need any assistance, call us."

Most men inject themselves easily. It is rare that a patient calls with a problem.

There is no way a patient can hurt himself with such a small needle, no matter where he injects. That's one worry that many patients have. The needle is so fine that most men will not notice any pain, especially if they are doing the injecting themselves. They are always telling me, "I didn't even feel it, Doc. It's amazing! I felt it more when you did it."

Common Worries

These are some common worries that my patients raise:

1. *What if I inject myself in the wrong place?*

If the injection is done incorrectly—for example, injected underneath the skin or injected in the urethra—you will simply not get an erection. Slight bleeding from the urethra may occur when you urinate, but this subsides spontaneously. We recommend that you take no aspirin or aspirin-containing products for 24–48 hours if this occurs. We have never had a complication from a patient injecting the urethra since the needle is very small and very thin.

If you inject the skin or the tissues below the skin, then no erection occurs, and you may get swelling of the penis on the periphery. This goes away rapidly.

2. *What if I hit a vein?*

If you hit a vein, you will probably get a small black-and-blue mark, which will go away in a week to 10 days.

3. *What if I inject air?*

Injecting air has happened. Patients have injected a full syringe of air into the penis, thinking that the syringe was full. What happens is that the air gets absorbed in the circulation, since it is only a 1 cc volume. It then gets carried to the right side of the heart through the venous system, and from the right side of the heart it goes to the lung, where it evaporates. It is the same principle with intravenous lines, where we often have air introduced through the I.V. line and on to the right heart and to the lung, where it is evaporated.

Injecting air is dangerous only if it is injected *directly* into an artery that leads to a major organ such as the heart or brain. There is no such artery in the penis.

4. *Will it hurt?*

The injection is quite painless due to the small size of the needle, even more so, patients tell us, when they are injecting themselves. Why? Because he is concentrating on where to do the injection, he's putting a little tension on the penis with his other hand, he's looking carefully, he's doing it slowly, and people always tell me that their second injection is less painful than their first injection for some reason. I think it's because they're doing the second themselves.

Of course, this is very subjective and there is great variability. Some people will put in the needle without thinking twice, but most men don't like the fact that they have to inject their penis. However, given the alternatives and given the fact that it's easy to do and quite painless, patients quickly become enthusiastic about the injection program. They get used to the idea and to the mechanics of injecting. Their perception of a needle injecting the penis is altered. Now they see it as, "Gee, it's like putting on a condom, just something I do before sex."

Sex is still spontaneous. Injecting is like taking one's clothes off before sex. That does not mean that sex is not spontaneous. Before sex, you give yourself an injection. Quite matter-of-fact. You still have to be aroused and excited; you still have to have the desire.

5. *What if it doesn't work?*

A lot of single men, particularly those who are divorced or widowed, and now a bit older and going out with a younger woman, are terrified of failing, especially on their first time and particularly if they had failed once before. They are sometimes totally absent from the lovemaking because they are monitoring their erections. How can you monitor your erection and at the same time pay attention to your partner? You just can't do two things at the same time.

In that group, they are concerned that they are not going to get an erection.

If, on top of that, the man does have some blockage of the arteries, some proven diminution of blood flow to the penis, then his anxieties will be even more elevated, and he's going to really depend on the injections.

What I recommend in that case is that he try it once alone at home, masturbating, with an erotic movie. See how it works. He may try it two or three times until he's sure it's reliable and that he can depend on it. Then he can try it the next time with a partner.

I tell them also to do it two or three times so that they become comfortable with injecting themselves, so they're not fumbling with needles and syringes. I tell them to prefill the syringes so that they are ready when needed. I tell them to excuse themselves, go to the bathroom, inject away from the bed so that the bed remains a place where romance is paramount. That keeps sex from becoming tied to the mechanical. You still need to have the arousal.

It might be better the first times to do it in your own setting, too, where there is no pressure and you can take your time. It's a matter of planning ahead, organizing, proceeding slowly and cautiously, and practicing. Practice is key, as with so many other skills.

Since the technique is quite easy, there is really not much to do. You just have to gain trust in the medication. (See Chapter 14 on possible side effects.)

Most men want to have sex two to four times a month. They are not looking to be studs, they just want to enjoy the simple pleasures that all human beings take for granted. This technique is definitely a valid option, if the patient would need to give himself only four injections in a month—which is far fewer than a diabetic gives.

Another advantage of pharmacological injections is that they may not be necessary all the time. Fifty percent of the patients in our Pharmacological Erection Program use the medication only intermittently, as they need it. They can start sex without it, knowing that there is something available, if needed, to guarantee an erection. If a man finds he doesn't want or need the medication, he can go ahead and have sex without it. It's not like getting an implant where you are destroying the remaining erectile capability of the penis in order to put in the implant. With injections, you don't destroy anything.

Some men will have sex a couple of times during a weekend without the injection, but on the third night, that Sunday night, they need the injection. Only 35% really need medication all the time, and 15% actually realize that just having the injection at home on hand as a security blanket makes them relax, and they are able to have sex without injections.

Regular followup visits are necessary to have the penis examined anywhere from every two months to a year, depending on how often injections are done. Some patients inject once a month, some two to three times a week.

The average age of my patients is in the 50s, and they range from 18 to 85. The average cost for pharmacological therapy is anywhere from $90 to $190 for 20 doses.

These medications are tremendous for young men who have a resistant psychological problem that has failed standard therapy and where the therapist doesn't know what else to do. We often work with therapists and will use combined sex therapy and injections. In this way, the patient gets immediate support and positive reinforcement with the injections.

We recommend that patients who have problems with injecting themselves see a therapist, also. This combination is extremely effective for younger patients who may have a psychological component in addition to a vascular problem.

If patients smoke, we tell them they must stop, because smoking is harmful to erectile function.

Cholesterol is important also, and we check this—not only total cholesterol but the ratio of good to bad cholesterol. If this ratio is bad, we recommend help with a cholesterol-lowering regimen.

So now you are on your own. You come back for followup treatments according to how many times you use the medication. We have patients who are eight to nine years on followup.

Theoretically, injections can continue for the rest of a man's life. Every patient presents with a varying set of needs as well as symptoms, which is why treatment must always be tailored to the individual. Even within the large group of men who are self-injecting, we have a wide range of personalities and challenges. Still, injection therapy manages to satisfy this spectrum of unique cases, such as this interesting case from our files. Mr. X is a salesman, 34 years old, who first came here last year, fairly thin, a pipe smoker with no past medical problems except for skull fracture when he got hit by a car 17 years before—but no injury to his pelvic area. Ten years ago, he developed problems with erections—difficulty getting an erection and then going soft after two to three minutes. His sleep study was abnormal, but his physical exam was unremarkable. He had already tried the oral drug, Yohimbine, but that didn't improve his erections. He seemed extremely anxious. It was hard for him to talk about his problem.

He was quite a puzzle. After several examinations it became clear that this man didn't have a psychological abnormality. Even though he had had the head trauma earlier, he says he had normal erections until 1981. The fact that he wasn't able to maintain an erection was suspicious for neurogenic dysfunction. This was our presumptive diagnosis, because this is what paraplegics and quadriplegics complain of. They are able to obtain but not maintain an erection. We also checked his hormones and everything came back normal.

We did a Duplex Ultrasonography, which showed he had good arterial blood flow. We immediately ruled out malfunction of the penile tissue that failed to trap the blood in the penis, such as a venous leak, and we ruled out an inflow problem. We felt it was not psychological because he did not respond to psychological therapy. We didn't need to pinpoint the problem's etiology any further than this, because treatment would be the same. And there wasn't any other neurological manifestation. He didn't have voiding problems, no sensitivity problems in the area of the penis.

He said to me: "What! You want me to do what, Doc? You're crazy!" when I told him about the injections. He was very nervous and told me he didn't want to do it. But then he did manage to try one injection in the office and got a tremendous erection. Now he said, "I can't wait to try this with my girlfriend."

Interestingly, Mr. X didn't respond to the milder PGE_1 (prostaglandin E_1). Despite several tries at home, he complained that he developed an ache. However, he responded well to papaverine/phentolamine. After several home trials with different mixtures of those drugs, the patient was entered into the Pharmacological Erection Program.

Mr. X started injecting himself, sometimes three to four times a week, with this combination of medication. He is extremely satisfied and very happy. Sometimes he reports four orgasms a night when he meets his girlfriend on weekends, and they have sex the whole weekend. He may inject himself two to three times during a weekend. We have warned him about in-

jecting so often, but he still winds up using the injections a lot—
he's a young man and bursting with desire.

Recently, he developed two nodules in the penis the size of a
beebee pellet. These represent scarring from the persistent injections. We think it is related to papaverine. He was urged to stop
injecting, but he didn't want to quit, so we got him to consider
other alternatives. He tried intercourse without injections without developing an erection. He tried intercourse with PGE_1 and
that didn't work either. Now, at our urging, he is contemplating
a penile implant, since he is very young, will need injections for
the rest of his life, and the implants are extremely successful and
satisfying in that situation. If he continues injecting, I think he
would develop more and more nodules and eventually his penis
would fail to respond to the injections. He comes for followup
once a month or so because he is injecting so often. This is a case
where the injections work so well that it is difficult to steer him
in another direction because he's so satisfied. We could simply
stop prescribing the medication, but that is the ultimate step. I
prefer to work along with patients as much as possible.

11

How to Self-Inject

We generally coach men to excuse themselves as they're making love or in the midst of foreplay and go to the bathroom to give themselves the injection at the root of the penis. After the patient is finished with the injection (which should take anywhere from 5 to 10 seconds), he returns to bed and continues lovemaking. As foreplay continues and goes into intercourse, the erection comes up very naturally, the rigidity improves, the man is able to maintain the erection longer, and after ejaculation there is partial detumescence, very much like a normal erection. It's not like an implant that stays up after ejaculation.

Fullness of the penis maintains itself usually for a couple of hours after injection, even after orgasm. If a man is restimulated or sex is started again, a second erection can occur.

Following is the procedure for self-injection.

Before you touch or clean the penis, you want to prepare your needle and syringes. I recommend that you have a couple of prefilled syringes, because you may be excited and aroused, and it may not be the best time to fill the syringe and play around with the needles.

First, you open your alcohol swab and have that ready. Hold

the medication bottle so that your fingers do not touch the rubber stopper through which the needle is inserted, and check the expiration date of the medication (Fig. 1). Using a circular motion, wipe off the top of the vial with the alcohol swab (Fig. 2).

Remove the needle cover. Don't allow the needle to touch anything prior to drawing the medication or before injecting (Fig. 3). Draw an amount of air equal to the amount of medication to be injected into the syringe. Push the needle through the center of the stopper. Push the air into the bottle (Fig. 4).

As shown in Figure 5, turn the bottle upside down and slowly draw the medication into the syringe. Tap the syringe gently to remove the bubbles.

Next, move the plunger in and out several times while gently tapping the syringe, thus removing all air bubbles.

Gently remove the needle from the vial and replace the cap. Remove the drawing needle and replace it with the 30g injecting needle.* Loosen the protective cap and place the filled syringe within easy reach prior to injecting (Fig. 7).

When everything is ready and your syringe is uncapped and the cap is replaced loosely on the needle, you then go into a comfortable position for the injection. If you're right-handed, you're going to put your left thigh on top of the sink counter. And your right leg totally extended touching the ground so you're half sitting, half standing.

Use the injection site illustrated in Figure 8. This area is designated on the drawing with crosshatch marks.

With the penis in that position, you take the alcohol swab and wipe the side of the penis near the base. With thumb and index finger you hold the head of the penis—only the head, none of the foreskin (if uncircumcised, you push the foreskin down).

---

*Also available are syringes armed with 29g needles which can serve to both draw and inject medication. In this case, there is no need to replace the needle.

Holding the head only, not the skin, pull until the penis is totally straight; pull it toward your left knee, positioning it along your inner thigh. Thus, you pull OUT—STRAIGHT DOWN toward the left knee. Maintain traction on the head after cleaning the side of the penis (Fig. 9).

Patients report that the closer they get to the base of the penis, the better the erection. Half of the penis is buried in the body; therefore, you want to make sure that you inject close to the base, that medication goes both towards the tip of the penis and towards the back of the patient. (However, to prevent scarring and to allow an area to heal, patients are instructed to vary the site of the injections along the shaft and on either side of the penis.)

Grasp the syringe between the thumb and middle finger like a pen. Place the needle on the site of injection at a 90° angle. Push in the needle gently but firmly all the way to the brown hub (Fig. 10). You want to inject toward the back of the penis and the side rather than underneath, or the belly, where the urethra is. But if you inject the urethra, don't worry. You just will not get an erection. But there's no way that you can hurt yourself. You can get a black and blue mark. In the beginning, patients do sometimes get those.

Shift your finger so that your index finger or your thumb can push in the plunger. Push in the medication slowly—over eight to 10 seconds (Fig.11).

Remove the needle and apply pressure with your index finger on the injection site and your thumb on the opposite side of the penis. Apply pressure for about two minutes (Fig. 12).

Actually, the hardest thing about injecting the penis is not the injection itself. The hardest thing is holding the penis for 30 seconds to two minutes after the injection at the spot where the needle went in so that you will not get a black and blue mark. Usually, a black and blue mark is the size of a beebee; it's very small and insignificant.

Injection Step by Step

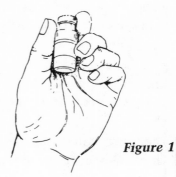

Figure 1

1. Hold the medication bottle so that your fingers do not touch the rubber stopper through which the needle is inserted. Check expiration date of medication.

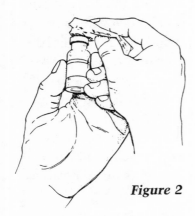

Figure 2

2. Using a circular motion, wipe off the top of the vial with an alcohol swab.

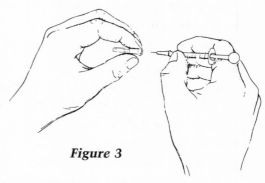

Figure 3

3. Remove the needle cover. Do not allow the needle to touch anything prior to drawing the medication or before injecting.

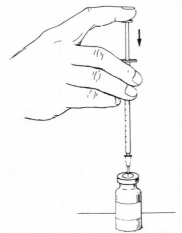

Figure 4

4. Draw an amount of air equal to the amount of medication to be injected into the syringe. Push the needle through the center of the stopper. Push the air into the bottle.

5. Turn the bottle and syringe upside down. Slowly draw the medication into the syringe. Tap the syringe gently to remove the bubbles.

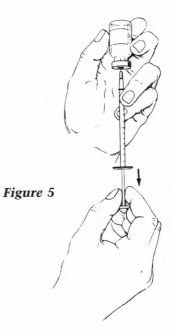

Figure 5

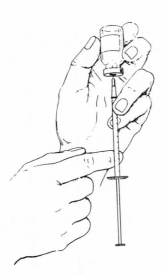

Figure 6

6. Move the plunger in and out several times while gently tapping the syringe, thus removing all air bubbles.

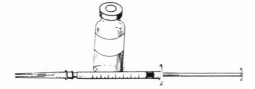

Figure 7

7. Gently remove the needle from the vial and replace the cap on it. Remove the drawing needle and replace with the 30g injecting needle. (If the syringe with the 29g needle is used, this step is unnecessary.) Loosen the protective cap and place the filled syringe within easy reach.

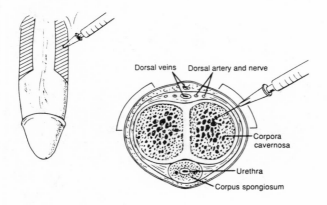

Dorsal veins   Dorsal artery and nerve

Corpora cavernosa

Urethra

Corpus spongiosum

Figure 8

8. Use injection site as illustrated. This area is designated on the drawing with crosshatch marks.

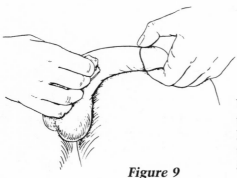

9. Locate the area of injection. Wipe with an alcohol swab. Grasp the head of the penis—not the skin. Position the penis along your inner thigh. Maintain traction on the head after cleaning the side of the penis.

Figure 9

10. Grasp the syringe between the thumb and middle finger like a pen. Place the needle on the site of injection at a 90° angle. Push the needle in gently but firmly all the way to the brown hub.

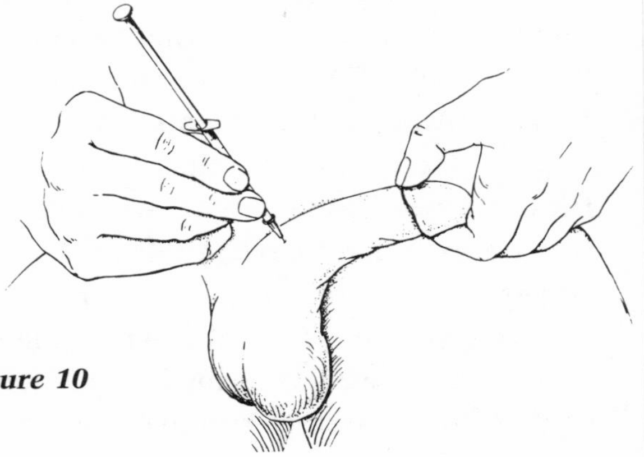

Figure 10

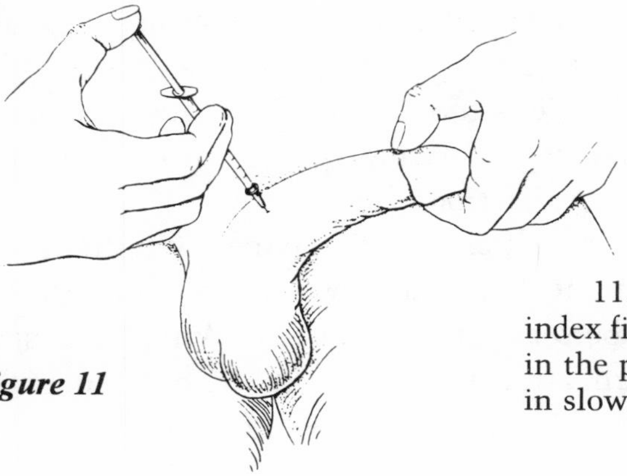

Figure 11

11. Shift your finger so that your index finger or your thumb can push in the plunger. Push the medication in slowly—over 8 to 10 seconds.

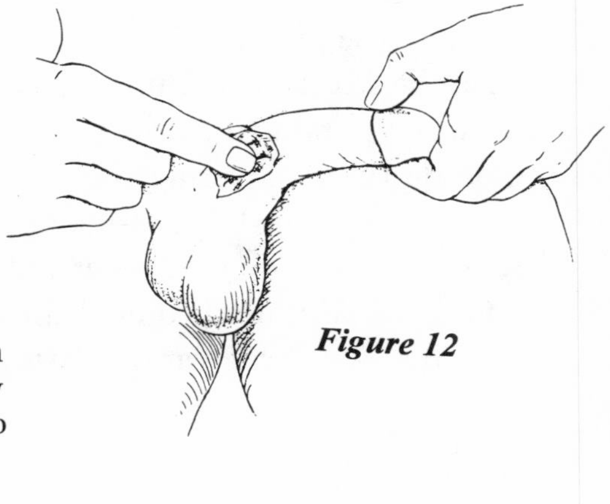

12. Remove the needle. Apply pressure with your index finger on the injection site and your thumb on the opposite side of the penis. Apply pressure for about 30 seconds to two minutes.

Figure 12

As one becomes more practiced in this procedure, it becomes second nature. Men don't even think about doing it anymore; they know exactly what to do and they do it quite rapidly. It's very easy. The key is to prepare, to set yourself up. Be comfortable. And practice, practice, practice.

You should have a couple of syringes prefilled because sometimes the needle will either fall off or you get a little nervous, so this way you don't have to refill the syringe. These syringes can be kept for a couple of weeks prefilled and refrigerated.

The Needles: The thinnest needle is a 30-gauge needle, and that's the one we feel is the best. Unfortunately, it's so thin you cannot fill the syringe through that needle because the lumen is so small. So you fill with the needle that comes with the syringe, discard that needle, and get yourself a fresh, 30-gauge needle. It's longer so it goes right to the center of the penis. Some patients feel that switching the needle is too much of an inconvenience and prefer to use the thicker 29g needle which can be used to both draw and inject the medication.

Each man injects a little differently. Some men will first try intercourse without it and if they find they are successful, they won't use it. It is always better to start without it. Why? Because if the penis is partially firm after stimulation, it is easier to inject than a flaccid, small penis. I always recommend that a man start foreplay first.

I also tell men to put a little tension on the penis by pulling it when they inject. Why? Because when they release the penis, then the stretchable lining—the corpora, or the tunica albuginea of the corporal body, which is the thick fascia that makes up the erectile tissue covering the inner elastic part of the penis that gets engorged with blood—squeezes the injection hole when you let go of it. So you get less of a black and blue mark; sometimes, you don't even need to hold the penis afterward.

Men will have varying reactions and practices:

1. Some men have told me: "If I start too early, it won't work."
2. Some men find that they need to take the medication out of the refrigerator (if it's the type that needs refrigeration), draw it into the syringe, and leave it out for about half an hour before they inject. They find if it's warmer it works better. (If it is prostaglandin E_1, it needs to be kept refrigerated; if it is papaverine/phentolamine, it does not.)
3. Some men find that if they stand up for five to 10 minutes after the injection, they will get a better erection. In these cases, they will inject themselves before foreplay.

The important thing about all this is that I encourage people to try different options, whatever they are most comfortable with and works best for them.

In addition, I tell men: You still need to be intimate, you still need to be excited. This is not a substitute. This is not a purely chemical erection. We have animal data that show you need nerve stimulation to enhance the pharmacologically induced erection. We have clinical investigation data that show that if you are erotically excited, your erection will be better. So, if you're very tired, or if you're not excited, or you don't want to have sex, you're not going to get a great erection. That's important to remember, because sometimes men expect that the medication is going to overcome a lack of interest or overcome fatigue. And it won't.

12

Three Cases of Injection Therapy

Generally speaking, after we do the screening and men get a response, we make the overall diagnosis of vascular erectile dysfunction, where appropriate. This covers a lot of possible causes. It could be that there's not enough inflow in the penis, or it could be that the muscle in the penis is not trapping blood in the penis, but basically it's due to a *biochemical* problem, possibly a decrease in the elastic fibers of the penis, or abnormal secretion of a chemical such as nitric oxide. The causes of the biochemical disturbance are frequently atherosclerosis and cholesterol—in other words, a vascular/arteriogenic problem.

Twelve years before he came to me, Mr. P tried to have sex with his fiancée and failed. They still went on to marry, but in their entire 12 years of marriage did not succeed in having intercourse, although he continued to have orgasm and ejaculation.

This isn't unusual. While the penis may remain soft, a man is often able to have both orgasm and ejaculation. Ironically, this contributes to the long wait before a man seeks treatment, because he continues to have pleasure without the erection.

In these 12 years, Mr. P became convinced of two things: First, that his problem was psychological, and second, if it *did* turn out to be physical, then the only possible cure was surgery. (Actually, this was the case in the '50s and '60s, but not anymore.)

He pursued sex therapy for two years without results. Since he didn't want surgery, at that point he gave up hope of having an erection. Finally, he came to our Unit when his family doctor retired and he went to see a new internist for a general checkup.

Mr. P always came alone to the Erectile Dysfunction Unit, and always had a sporty look. He wore expensive-casual clothes and was well groomed. He talked a lot to everyone, talked to my secretaries, talked to my assistant. He looked at our brochure and corrected it. He was that type of guy—fully involved and fully committed to his treatment and finding out what was wrong with him.

He was a bit overweight. Otherwise, everything looked good. He was diabetic and on insulin. We did the Duplex test and documented that his arteries were not dilating well, so his penile blood flow wasn't good. Then I gave him a test injection and he achieved a partial erection. The diagnosis: arteriogenic dysfunction, which was consistent with his other problem—blocked coronary arteries.

He started on prostaglandin E_1, which is the mildest of the erection drugs. I gave him several syringes of the drug to try at home, and he came back the following week to tell me, with tears running down his face, that he had successfully made love with penetration for the first time in 12 years.

That to me is testimonial to what today's treatment can do.

Medications, of course, aren't the total answer to everything. There are many elements involved in an erection, particularly the psychological and one's own physical state.

However, the pharmacological approach is an effective treatment because it does not interfere with the workings of a natural erection. It *enhances* it. There is nothing mechanical about it.

Then there was Mr. M, tall, 69 years old, with a light tan, gray hair combed back, well dressed, self-assured, a successful executive. He didn't speak much at first. He felt his sexual interest was "normal"; he preferred females. Morning erections were rare.

He described that with masturbation he had ejaculation with a soft penis. I consider that one of the key signals for organic dysfunction.

His erections first faltered at age 40! He had family problems at the time, so he thought it was psychological. When he was 56, he remarried and had a good sexual life, but his erections were never what they were before age 40. He had occasional penetration; sometimes his penis was rigid enough, sometimes not, and sometimes it lacked maintaining ability.

Risk factors included a long history of hypertension. Mr. M was on several medications for that. His cholesterol level was normal. He had a history of tobacco smoking, but had stopped 35 years ago. His second wife, who was younger than he, was keenly disappointed in his lack of performance. Given the fact that he looked healthy and younger than his stated age, she felt cheated. Like, why me? Why couldn't I find a man who could have sex like everybody else?

We did the first injection in the office and Mr. M developed a fairly rigid erection with a mixture of papaverine/phentolamine, which is our standard test dose. The erection lasted about 30 minutes. He came back 20 days later for his first self-injection with a special mixture of papaverine and PGE_1. He had no problem injecting himself. He came only for two visits, and required only one home trial with two choices of medication, which we gave him on his second visit. He told us the better one had the higher dose of PGE_1, and he has been on that dose ever since. He came back just for followup and it's been seven months since I last saw him.

He said that he is thrilled because now he can *relax*; he

knows he is going to have an erection. He reports that 50% of the time he can have intercourse without the shots, and that his erections are better. He also uses a ring to enhance his erection, and says he can penetrate with the ring alone without injections. (This is a ring from the Osbon Erec Aid Vacuum, a device that comes with a vacuum pump and serves to trap the blood in the penis once the vacuum pump is activated.) The other 50% of the time, he is unable to maintain an erection long enough for intercourse and it is those times that he injects himself. So he uses injections about three to four times a month.

That is the advantage of injections, as opposed to a theoretical pill or patch. You deliver the drug when you want it. The response is immediate. Therefore, you can first try sex without it. You don't have to take a pill one to two hours ahead of time whenever you want to have sex. If you rely on a pill and have to wait half an hour to an hour, your partner is going to be furious or bored by that time and she's going to say forget it. Let's do it another night.

Dr. Q is a 61-year-old dentist. He developed erectile dysfunction five years ago. He had high cholesterol and a history of blocked arteries in the heart, so it made sense that he would have blocked arteries in the penis as well. Combine tobacco, four packs a day for 35 years, and his age. Put that together with ejaculation with a soft penis and occasional penetration without maintaining ability, and I know it is going to be a physical problem.

He received his first injection with PGE_1 and developed a great erection. That same day, because he was a dentist and knew how to handle needles, we gave him three samples of different doses of PGE_1—5, 6, and 7 mcg. He used them at home, said they were great, came back, entered the Pharmacological Erection Program, and has been using the medication steadily since. We saw him eight months later and gave him two bottles of medication because he wants one for his country home and one for his city home.

Regardless of age, background, and education, patients are often repelled by the vacuum device, but love the injections. They would prefer a pill, if one were available, but after I explain to them about the drawbacks of a pill, they are happy with the injections.

If a young patient is contemplating a penile implant, we put him on injections temporarily so we can see if he has a psychological problem. We try to get a feeling if his problem is related to performance anxiety or is physical. If it is psychological, he'll do well on injections because he'll prove himself with his partner and the next time he makes love, he will not have to prove himself. He just has to have fun while having sex and eventually can wean himself off injections.

13

Romance

I know that these new potency treatments can be regarded as a "quick fix." When I see a man who is intimate with his wife and everything is fine between them, but he definitely has a vascular problem, then I zero in on the quick fix because that is what will serve him best. But when I see that intimacy is missing, that is hard for me to ignore.

As a society, we are so busy with our work or play that we are always actively doing something. We are seldom intimate, just being with somebody in a way that leads naturally to intimacy. That is one thing that is hard to tell patients. Men come to me wanting the quick fix. They don't want to spend time putting back intimacy, putting all the lovey dovey things back into their relationship. They want an erection—period!

When I tell them, "This medication works, but if you also have the intimacy, it will work even better, and maybe you won't even need drugs after a while," they don't like to hear that. "My wife is not really into that kind of stuff, anyway," they argue. I'm sure a lot of wives would be surprised to hear it!

However, men don't come to me for counseling, and they know I'm not professionally qualified to help them work on intimacy per se. A man sitting across my desk generally just wants to know why his penis is not getting hard and how to make it get hard again. At the same time, an erection is a complicated event that depends on hormones, blood flow, and nerves; emotional stimulation definitely affects all those factors.

When I point out that it could be very exciting when a wife starts expressing herself sexually, some don't believe it. They've been with me half an hour and here I am telling them that their wife is as excited about sex as they are. And they've been with their wives for 35 years, so they know better—that's how they feel. What could this guy possibly be telling me?

Some time ago a letter to the "Playboy Magazine Adviser" asked: What is the most erogenous organ in the human body? Their answer surprised me, considering the focus of that magazine: the brain. This is a message I try to get across along with the purely physical treatments that medicine can offer today.

Women's Reactions to Injections

Some women get turned off by penile injections, but I believe even more are turned on. They get freed of worry about their husband's performance and can relax and enjoy sex. Of the men who come to see us, most of their mates are very supportive. They are also supportive because this is "his thing, he's taking care of it. If he's happy, I'm happy." They are also happy because, again, it provides all the physical and emotional benefits of a natural erection.

It doesn't bother many couples to have the injection at the bedside. Some accept it with a lot of humor.

It is also nice that once the injection is done, then the only thing to do is to have sex rather than to inflate an implant or use a pump.

The kit of medication wouldn't fit in a man's suit pocket, but it doesn't have to. You don't have to have the whole kit with you. We offer a little plastic case that can hold two or three prefilled syringes and that can fit in a pocket. So it's not obtrusive and it's easy to transport.

Do you want to get your mate involved? The answer to this is not cut-and-dried. Each couple is different. Some wives want to know about everything their husband is doing. Some don't particularly want to know.

Also, this varies according to how relaxed your mate is about sex. Some women are very relaxed; some are very embarrassed and would never come to the office with their husbands. Some women will send me their regards and some husbands never talk about their wives. But these men come back, so that's how I know that their mates must be satisfied, too. I'd say about 60–75% of all patients on the injection program keep coming back for medication for their injections.

Very rarely will a woman do the injecting. Most men do it themselves, except for the spinal-cord injured, the quadriplegics; their wives will often learn to inject them. For most men, it's really like brushing their teeth or putting on a condom. Most men put on their own condoms and it's part of their hygiene. Similarly, a diabetic wouldn't expect his wife to give him his insulin injections, unless he were incapacitated.

Women can pretty well rest easy once their mate is going for treatment and getting the medications. She doesn't have to worry too much about anything that she has to do. She can just be sexy.

Recently, one of my patients told me: "I don't see my girlfriend that often." (He's 71 years old.) "I see her two weekends a month. We make love Friday, we make love Saturday, and then Sunday I can't get it up. So I use the injection on Sunday. That's the only time I use it, Doc. And, I can have an erection for two hours with the injection. It's great. My partner loves it. She has five to six orgasms!"

So people are different and make their own adjustment.

(The reason he could have erections two days in a row and not the third is that as a man gets older, he doesn't recover as quickly and needs more and more time to get have an erection and ejaculation.)

What to Expect from Sexual Life with Injections

The responses are very positive. Men feel great. They feel manly again. A lot of men get their erection on the initial test and they want to leave the office with the erection.

"Will it last until I get home? Will it last until tonight?" Almost everybody asks me that.

They don't want to waste it. They say, "Gee, I haven't had an erection in 14 years; I gotta use this one!"

The fact that a man has gone without an erection for a long time doesn't mean that he can't have one again.

I would say you can ordinarily expect a normal life with pharmacological injections—maybe even better than normal because your erections will be more predictable. They will last longer, and that makes sex even better than normal.

14

Questions and Answers About Injections and the Medications

Following are some of the questions most asked about the injection treatment for Erectile Dysfunction.

Who Uses This Type of Treatment?

A wide range of men use injections to obtain erections. Generally, they are active and would like to remain sexually active as well. Men who are reluctant to have surgery find injections a good alternative.

Who Is a Candidate for the Pharmacological Injections?

In general, men who suffer from erectile dysfunction and who obtain erections with injections are candidates for this treatment. Contraindications to penile injections include: sickle cell disease, poor manual dexterity or poor vision, and an inability or unwillingness to follow instructions, creating potential for misuse or abuse.

How Long Have the Medications Been Used for This Purpose?

Papaverine and phentolamine have been used for stimulating erections since 1983. PGE_1 has been used only for the last three to four years.

How Safe Are These Medications?

They are extremely safe, although, like any medications, they do have side effects. Papaverine has been used for over 20 years for dilation of the arteries in the heart as well as for Alzheimer's disease and multiple sclerosis. Radiologists use papaverine during radiological procedures involving the arteries. One of the toxic effects reported with papaverine is a skipped heartbeat or abnormal conduction in the heart. This usually occurs when large doses are given. Cardiologists and surgeons have used up to 120 mg of papaverine intravenously every three hours without toxic effects. The usual dosage in the penis is 30 mg or less. Therefore, with the amount of papaverine we use, we are well under toxic dose levels.

Phentolamine, also used for a long time, lowers the blood pressure when given in higher doses. It can also produce heartbeat irregularities, diarrhea, and abdominal discomfort. This medication was used in the past, in 5 mg doses, to uncover tumors of the adrenal glands. The dose used in the penis is 0.5 mg to 1 mg, again well away from toxic dose levels.

Prostaglandin E_1 is by far the safest of all drugs we use. It is an excellent medication for dilation of the arteries, and is used in high doses in premature babies with cardiac malformations. PGE_1 is rapidly metabolized in the lungs should it leak from the penis. The dose used for erections is minute, anywhere from five to 40 micrograms.

WHAT ARE THE POTENTIAL SIDE EFFECTS?

Very little can go wrong. Even if you inject air, nothing will happen. Some men have done that because they don't see that the fluid is not going into the syringe. Because the volume is small, the air goes to the veins, which go to the right side of the heart and on to the lungs. And from the lungs all the air evaporates into the atmosphere. A lot of people think that air injected into the veins will go to the brain, but this isn't the case.

Basically, side effects break down into two categories. There are those produced whenever a needle is stuck into one's body: a small bruise may develop at the site over time, a small nodule or lump may develop if the same site is injected again and again. Rarely, scarring of the inner body of the penis might occur. Plaque can develop at the site of the injection.

The scarring and plaque of Peyronie's disease can be mistaken for an injection side effect. Peyronie's disease is an inflammatory condition of unknown cause. This disease can manifest itself by curvature, pain, and induration of the erectile bodies. Erections can worsen the discomfort and accentuate the curvature. An hourglass or constrictive deformity may also be noted when the penis is erect. Decreased rigidity of erection as well as shortening of the penis may be noted. More subtly, the first manifestation of Peyronie's disease may be decreased inability to maintain an erection. Pain and curvature may appear much later (six months).

So let's say the patient is injecting himself. The penis then develops a curvature. He may blame it on the medication, when actually it is the Peyronie's disease that is progressing. After a lot of injections, usually with papaverine, over a long period of time, it is possible for nodules to develop. Some people (about 10%) have this reaction, but most do not. This scarring and fibrosis could be due to the repeated injections or medication. However, usually it is the manifestation of Peyronie's disease.

If I see someone getting a plaque, they have to stop injecting since this could make the plaque worse. Some men say, "I'm not going to get an implant. And I'm not going to do anything else. So I'd like to keep injecting." I tell them: There is no way to prevent plaque from occurring if injections are continued.

However, now that we're using thin needles and smaller doses of papaverine or PGE_1 fewer people get plaque. This has rarely been a problem.

The second category of side effects are those produced by the medications. Papaverine and phentolamine may produce a painful, sustained, prolonged erection, known as priapism. This occurs mostly in the beginning when a doctor is attempting to adjust the medication dose to suit that particular patient. Priapism (an erection lasting longer than four hours) requires immediate medical attention. It is easy to reverse when treated early.

Other side effects, which are rare, include dizziness or headache. Even less frequently is an increase in liver enzymes usually associated with papaverine. Prostaglandin E_1 is safer, as it rarely produces priapism or liver enzyme abnormalities. A natural product of the body, PGE_1 is broken down locally by enzymes present in the penis. One possible side-effect of PGE_1 is a slight, dull ache in the penis. This usually subsides after about 15 minutes.

What If I Inject the Wrong Place?

You could inject into the urethra; you won't get an erection. You could inject into a vein; you'll get a black and blue mark on the penis and won't get an erection.

What's the Most Serious Thing That Can Happen?

The most serious thing that can go wrong is to have a *prolonged erection*. That is why the first two injections are done in the office. So we see how strong a dose you need.

Is There Any Danger from Use of the Needles?

It is better to throw away the needle each time, but you could reuse the needle if you like. Diabetics now are reusing their needles, and it's OK for them to do it. I know of diabetics who use one needle 15 times to save money. It just must be kept clean, of course. The needle is drawing the medication into the syringe and then hitting the skin where there are some bacteria, but the alcohol swab kills everything. The needle goes on into the fatty tissue and blood vessels. The medication gets pushed through the needle and then the needle is withdrawn. If it is capped, there shouldn't be any bacteria. Even if there are bacteria injected into the skin, the white cells will destroy them right away. So unless someone is immunosuppressed, nothing will happen. You don't have to wipe the needle with alcohol afterward.

However, we do recommend that you switch to a *new needle* each time. There are two reasons for that. One, you don't want to put any blood back into the bottle. And two, there can be a little clot of blood in the lumen of the syringe, which would prevent you from injecting. Actually, needles and syringes are so cheap, that it is just as well to change them each time.

IS THE INJECTION PAINFUL?

Over 90% of our patients tell us they are surprised at how painless the injections are. Also, since the needle hole is very tiny, little bruising or bleeding occurs.

HOW EXPENSIVE IS THE MEDICATION?

The approximate cost of a two-month supply of papaverine and phentolamine with syringe and needles begins at $115. Prostaglandin E_1 comes in 10, 20, 30, and 40 mcg per cc concentration, and a 10-cc bottle at 10 mcg per cc concentration starts at $90, including syringes and needles.

HOW OFTEN CAN I USE INJECTIONS?

The number of injections is not to exceed 10 per month. We recommend injections be spaced evenly. Also, the site of injection should alternate between left and right side of the penis.

DOES IT WORK?

The pharmacological treatment has been successful in producing erections in over 80% of the patients seen at the Erectile Dysfunction Unit. This erection is more than adequate to perform intercourse. The rest of the patients in whom injections have no effect are candidates for other forms of treatment.

How Long Before Medications Start to Work?

An erection occurs anywhere from 10 to 20 minutes following injection. Generally, PGE_1 works slightly faster than papaverine/phentolamine. A better erection is usually obtained with the addition of foreplay. Some men require a 30-minute wait before obtaining a fully rigid erection. In general, the amount of time it takes to obtain an erection is a correlate of the extent of arterial blockage.

How Long Will the Erection Be Maintained?

Anywhere from 20 minutes to an hour and a half is considered a successful result.

How Long Before the Medication Expires?

Papaverine/phentolamine is effective for 60 days. Dr. Lloyd Allen of the University of Oklahoma College of Pharmacy studied the stability of the mixture. He showed that when stored in a refrigerated temperature of 40° Fahrenheit, papaverine lost less than 3% of its activity and phentolamine less than 7%. Stored at room temperature (77° Fahrenheit), papaverine lost less than 3% of activity and phentolamine less than 9% over a 60-day period. PGE_1 must be kept refrigerated at 42° Fahrenheit and will last for four months.

Do Pharmacological Erections Cure the Arterial Blockage?

Injections do not cure or reverse blockage of the arteries. They allow one to obtain an erection without the need of surgery or a penile prosthesis. Furthermore, injections may not continue to work, especially if the condition (high cholesterol, high blood pressure, etc.) continues to affect the penile arteries. Tobacco smoking will also affect erectile function and may worsen the atherosclerosis of the penile arteries to the point where injections may not work.

CAN I STILL HAVE AN ORGASM?

Erections produced by injections do not interfere with orgasm. If you were able to have an orgasm without the injections, you will continue to do so on injections.

NO REACTIONS AT ALL?

If there is no reaction at all to the injection, that usually indicates that the medication was put below the skin and not into the body of the penis.

CAN I INJECT MORE THAN ONCE A NIGHT?

It's very important not to inject twice in one night. If it doesn't work once, forget it. Try it again tomorrow. The reason is that you don't know exactly where that medication is. And that's when people may get into problems if they develop a prolonged erection after a second injection in a short period of time.

A prolonged erection is dangerous. When it is prolonged and rock-hard, the arteries that feed and nurture the penis are no longer able to carry nutrients and oxygen into the penis, because the pressure in the penis is higher than the pressure generated from the heart. Therefore, there is no flow of blood into it and the muscles in the penis start becoming anoxic (lacking in oxygen).

Lactic acid formation makes things worse and the tissue starts dying. Cells die. The tissue loses its elasticity and then the patient doesn't respond to injections anymore.

This can happen after probably 12 hours of a prolonged erection. I've seen people with prolonged, rock-hard erections for 24 hours and nothing happened, but I think some of these changes start to occur between 12 and 24 hours.

INADEQUATE RESPONSE?

You've got the dose right, but still you don't respond? That rarely happens. The medications are quite reliable. The patients who complain that they are erratic are generally the spinal-injured men, who can have erratic responses. I don't know why. You could have two spinal-cord injured men, both at the level of T4-5-T6. One will get an excellent erection with only 0.2 cc of papaverine, and the other needs 60 mg—or 2 cc—of papaverine—10 times the dose. Paraplegics usually respond better to papaverine.

WHAT ABOUT TOO FREQUENT APPLICATIONS?

We warn men about scar tissue formation, and we suggest that they alternate sides for injections. Keep a log sheet. The maximum frequency would be two to three times a week.

WHAT DOES THE FOOD AND DRUG ADMINISTRATION (FDA) SAY ABOUT THESE MEDICATIONS?

There is no disclaimer or warning on the phentolamine or prostaglandin E_1 bottles saying they shouldn't be used for penile injections. There is a disclaimer on the bottle for papaverine. Although papaverine is approved by the FDA for use in the human body, the manufacturer states that "Papaverine hydrochloride is not indicated for the treatment of impotence by intracorporal injections." However, there were no clinical trials.

The Physician's Desk Reference does not indicate that you can use these medications for injection into the penis. So this is a non-indicated, but accepted, use of these medications. Patients need to keep in mind that they are not approved by the FDA for this use. However, after widespread use of these medications for erectile dysfunction throughout the world, there seem to be no serious side effects of the medications used in this way.

Good clinical trials with long-term followups are needed to meet the requirement of the FDA in this regard. Until then, there will always be some degree of uncertainty. We know that at the small doses used and in the appropriate patient, the medication seems to be safe and effective.

We are looking at ways to change this FDA situation. Given all the complications related to silicon breast implants, injection therapy has become an attractive alternative to penile implants in many cases. As more baby boomers age and reach 50–55, we'll see a lot of changes in these areas, I'm sure.

WHAT ABOUT INSURANCE?

Some insurance companies don't recognize erection problems as medical. Many still regard this as a "cosmetic" problem, so they don't reimburse for treatment. Another difficulty is that many men with this problem work in companies where all their insurance papers go through company channels, so that means others in the company can find out what is going on with them sexually, and their privacy is compromised.

MYTHS TO OUTGROW

There are a few common myths about penile injections. One is that the penis is highly sensitive and, therefore, injecting will be terribly painful. (It is not and it isn't.) Also, many men assume the injections must be made into the tip or into the urethra, which is not true. It is also a myth that injections will frighten away their sexual partners. And, finally, too many men think injections will prove to be a quick fix that will cure everything that is wrong with a relationship. This last myth dies especially hard. There are many factors affecting a relationship, and erectile dysfunction, while important, may be just one of many.

CAN MY PARTNER HELP?

As for the question of the reaction of sexual partners, in most instances, I find them to be both helpful and interested.

Some men actually come to see me because their mate has heard about injection therapy and insists that they investigate. These men often bring along their sexual partner, and that gives me a feel for the existing relationship. That relationship is the foundation for a good erection.

Maybe on the theory that if *one* interested helper is good, two could be even better, one man, Mr. R, showed up with his wife and his mistress. He liked to eat—and was diabetic—but wouldn't give up eating rich food. As you can imagine, he was greatly overweight. He smoked, but didn't drink. This was his second wife to whom he'd been married for eight years. She and his ladyfriend were best friends. It was a very complicated picture. This man marched to his own drum.

Because of his overweight, the wife and the mistress had to do the injection for him. I taught all three how to do the injections in the same room at the same time. They thought it was very funny because I didn't know whom to look at. They assumed that was because I was nervous, but actually I'm just not accustomed to teaching a "class" in self-injections. However, they were all animated and interested, and they picked up the technique quickly. They're probably used to shocking people with their happy ménage-à-trois.

In addition to counseling men to stop smoking, we also urge men who are overweight to lose pounds. With Mr. R, I was adamant, not just to aid his erections and the injecting procedure, but to help him with his diabetes.

Then there was one man, Mr. K, who brought his wife for the initial consultation, but they fought the entire time. He'd been living on high-fat food for at least 30 years, he was greatly overweight, and he smoked. He hadn't had intercourse for nine years. (She said nine, he said four, and they argued over that for 10 minutes.) He wanted her to leave while I took down the history, but she refused and corrected his answers, although the experience is basically foreign to women. She did leave during the physical exam and the various tests. Then, when I was ready to give my diagnosis, she rejoined us.

When she heard that his reduced erections were probably due to an unhealthy diet and smoking, she got livid. She blasted him for not seeing a doctor long ago. He wasn't concerned about her, she said. Maybe if he had been, he wouldn't have this problem. All during this tirade, Mr. K tried to talk to me about football!

Most of the time when men have trouble talking about their problems with erections or in handling injections, their mates can be a big help.

WHAT ABOUT INTIMACY—IS IT NECESSARY?

Intimacy may be the most important factor in building and maintaining a good sexual relationship and good sexual functioning. It is essential to bring the nerves—which are stimulated by the emotions—into the sex act so as to enhance the erection and enrich the entire experience. Perhaps the old adage, "Love conquers all" is truer than we think and is the foundation for resolving erectile problems. Intimacy gives a real boost to a man's erection.

15

Prevention of Potency Problems

There are a number of factors that, in our experience, are likely to have a strong influence on potency. These factors are important in general health problems, as well, and every individual would do well to make them a part of his or her lifestyle. Any disease states or habits associated with atherosclerosis, decreased lumen of blood vessels, and decreased blood flow, such as high cholesterol blood levels, high blood pressure, and tobacco smoking, are risk factors for developing erection problems.

High-Fat Diet and High Serum-Cholesterol Levels

There are no epidemiological studies linking high-fat diets or high serum-cholesterol levels with erection problems. However, at The New York Hospital–Cornell Medical Center we are studying decreasing serum-cholesterol level and its connection with erectile function. There are some interesting papers in the literature that show that the blockage of arteries at the level of the retinal vessels does improve with lowering of cholesterol.

I believe that all patients should know their cholesterol level.

It should be less than 200 with an HDL of greater than 45 for men (greater than 55 for females). A diet high in polyunsaturated fats maintains LDLs at a high level, which is undesirable. LDLs should be less than 125, with a ratio of HDL to total less than 2.5.

Athletes should know that steroids increase total cholesterol level and lower HDL cholesterol (the "good" cholesterol). Steroids also decrease serum testosterone levels and create infertility. So athletes should be aware of the dangerous side effects of these medications. There are many other side effects, as well.

High Blood Pressure

The best way to reduce hypertension is to lose weight, decrease salt intake to less than 2 grams a day, decrease alcohol consumption to less than 2 ounces a day. Reduce saturated fats. Increase intake of fruits and roughage. Learn and practice biofeedback techniques if blood pressure remains high. Do aerobic exercises. A deficiency in potassium, magnesium, and calcium may also be related to hypertension.

Overweight

There is a real incentive for overweight men to lose excess weight. Experts in erectile dysfunction believe that for every 35 pounds of weight loss by an obese person there is an apparent increase of penile length of approximately one inch. Obese men carry their weight at the level of their abdomen, a portion of which is above the penis and thus shortens the shaft of the penis. Losing weight is probably the best lengthening penile option available for men at present.

To keep potency alive, it is important to cultivate good exercise habits. It is important to exercise before meals, usually before the evening meal. Exercise tranquilizes and energizes, suppresses the appetite, and stimulates and makes the rest of the day more productive.

In addition to benefitting from an improved erectile response, men who exercise are less depressed, less hypochondriacal, have a better self-image, and generally display a better attitude toward life.

Care of the Penis

The penis is not just a muscle and it's also good for a man to realize it's not a steel pipe. It's a complicated hydraulic system that coordinates muscles, blood flow, nerves, and hormones. Very often, men tend to think of their penis in an erect state as being safe from any injury. That's a wrong concept.

Two things can happen that can irreversibly injure the penis.

The penis can fracture. This can occur when a man makes love to a woman from behind, sort of "doggy style." He will withdraw a little too much, then go back into the vagina, but as he goes back in, the penis drops a little, and instead of going straight into the vagina, the penis hits the pubic bone, which is just below the vagina. Men describe hearing a "snap," a cracking sound. Suddenly the penis loses the erection, and a huge hematoma— black and blue swelling—appears around the shaft of the penis. The penis goes totally flaccid and becomes swollen with a lot of blood below the skin. What has occurred is that a hole has been made in the shaft, in the lining of the penis. Actually, the hole looks like a bullet hole. The penis has a very thick tunica albuginea. The overlying skin is very loose, and that is where the hole is. So, when it bleeds, it is like when you get bumped on the head; you get a big lump. Moreover, the bleeding will continue.

This constitutes an emergency. The man needs to be treated immediately. He will need to be taken to the operating room, the hole must be found and then closed with stitches.

I had a patient who damaged his penis badly twice in this manner.

Another source of injury to the penis can arise from sports and exercise. There is a syndrome known as injury from a bicycle seat, but we see that only in professional bike racers who spend six hours a day on their bicycle seat, which is very narrow. These bikers have very little fat, they're extremely muscular. The bicycle seat hits the nerves going to the penis and damages the corporal bodies of the penis right at the root. We've had one Olympic bicycle champion as a patient.

Men can become impotent from trauma from the bicycle seat, but usually the ordinary bicycler will not run into this. The damage is reversible if a man stops bicycling. Since it is more of an injury to a nerve than to a vessel, once you remove the injury to the nerve, then the nerve grows back again.

The man who exercises vigorously doesn't need to wear special clothing. Just follow common sense. It may be good to wear a jock strap, but I don't think that's totally necessary because the detrusor muscles hold the testicles. This is different from breasts, which have no muscle tissue at all and need support in impact aerobics, whereas the penis is anchored.

16

Breakthroughs Ahead

Oral Medications

There have been a number of medicines that were thought to help with erections. One in particular is Yocon—or *yohimbine*. This comes in pill form, which in itself makes it attractive to many people.

Two adequate studies were done with yohimbine.* They both failed to show conclusively that yohimbine was helpful with erectile dysfunction. The first study, conducted by Dr. Alvaro Morales of the Department of Urology at Queens University in Kingston, Ontario showed that only 26% of the patients who took yohimbine reported reappearance of a full and sustained erection. The second study, in 1987, was performed by the same doctor and showed that 42% of the patients receiving yohimbine versus 27% receiving placebo had a positive response to the medication. However, when the data were statistically exam-

---

*Morales, A. *The Journal of Urology,* June, 1987. Is yohimbine effective in the treatment of organic impotence? Results of a controlled trial. Vol. 137, pp. 1168–1172.

ined, there was no statistical significance. The number of patients was not large enough to claim that placebo was not as good as yohimbine. They concluded that yohimbine showed a modest effectiveness at 18 mg per day for patients suffering from erectile dysfunction.

A lot of patients whom I see have tried yohimbine previously and it didn't work, or it made them jittery or nervous. The overall thinking is that yohimbine provides only modest results. Most likely, I think, as time passes, this drug will fall into disuse.

One of the oral medications currently being studied is oxytocin. Blood levels of oxytocin have been found to be increased after ejaculation, and infusions of oxytocin in dogs produced an erection and ejaculation. A group in LaJolla, California, is looking at the use of oxytocin as a nasal spray for treatment of impotence. No results are available, as yet.

Patches

Minoxidil and nitroglycerine have been used as patches to facilitate an erection. Dr. Giorgio Cavallini of the Department of Urology at the Hospital of Adria in Venetto, Italy, has tested minoxidil patch versus nitroglycerine patch versus a placebo patch.* His study was performed in 33 patients, and minoxidil proved to be more active than nitroglycerine and placebo in increasing diameter, rigidity, and arterial flow in the penis. It seems that the patients who benefitted most from this application were the neurogenically impotent patients. In addition, fewer side effects were noted with minoxidil than with nitroglycerine.

Patches have long proposed for the treatment of erectile dys-

---

*Cavallini, G. *The Journal of Urology,* July, 1991. Minoxidil versus nitroglycerin: A prospective double-blind controlled trial in transcutaneous erection facilitation for organic impotence. pp. 50–53.

function. However, any medication delivered in this fashion will be absorbed into the circulation and thus carried away from the desired site of action. If you put it on the penile skin, it will be absorbed and carried away from deeper blood vessels of the penis. Therefore, they are less effective than other methods.

Nitric Oxide

In the vast majority of men, erection problems can be traced to abnormal blood flow into the penis, as well as to a failure to trap and retain blood in the penis. The mechanism of blood trapping is well known, but no one knew how this event is initiated. Several chemicals were thought to relax the muscle cells in the penis so that blood flows in and remains trapped. (See Chapter 5, "How an Erection Happens.") However, after careful scrutiny, none of these chemicals was found to be effective in a consistent fashion.

Nitric oxide is secreted by the cells lining the blood vessels of several organs. Since the penis is made up of blood vessels, it seemed logical to assume that nitric oxide was also produced in the penis. This was recently demonstrated by Dr. Jacob Rajfer, professor of urology at the University of California in Los Angeles, who found that defects in the nitric oxide system of the penis account for the vast majority of impotence among American men.*

Nitric oxide is probably secreted by the nerves and sends a dilation message to the smooth muscle cells in the penis. The lining of the blood vessels in the penis also secrete nitric oxide, which diffuses to the smooth muscle cells and is followed by dilation.

---

*Rajfer, J. *The New England Journal of Medicine,* January, 1992. Nitric oxide as a mediator of relaxation of the corpus cavernosum in response to nonadrenergic, noncholinergic neurotransmission. pp. 90–94.

Linsidomine chlorhydrate, an antianginal drug, is believed to liberate nitric oxide from the walls of blood vessels. Just recently in some European settings, this medication was injected into the penis and seemed to cause an erection by releasing nitric oxide. These results are extremely promising since the drug uses the natural pathways of the erectile mechanism and could prove to be the ideal medication for penile injections in the future.*

Over the last seven years, thousands of men have been self-injecting medications at the root of the penis. These medications work by raising the nitric oxide levels and relaxing the smooth muscle cells. Thus, they bring on an erection that lasts half an hour or longer. Nitric oxide itself is unstable, difficult to synthesize, and impossible to store. Prostaglandin E_1, however, has been shown to raise nitric oxide levels in the penis and provide an erection.

How this discovery regarding nitric oxide will be utilized clinically in the future still remains to be seen. It could possibly one day lead to a removable patch to be placed on the penis to cause an erection.

I think nitric oxide will be a factor in the future. However, it should be emphasized that prostaglandin E_1 is hard to beat right now because it is almost everywhere in the body and there are enzymes to break it down everywhere. It is a natural chemical, naturally made in the body, and it is harmless. The major role in treatment of erectile dysfunction for the next five years, I believe, belongs to prostaglandin E_1.

---

*See Stief, C.G. et. al. (1992). Preliminary results with the nitric oxide donor linsidomine chlorhydrate in the treatment of human erectile dysfunction. *Journal of Urology, 148,* 1437–1440.

Angioplasty

Angioplasty of the penile arteries also looks like a possible break-through frontier for potency in the future. Penile arteries are much smaller than those in other areas of the body where such procedures are now done, but technology is progressing to where it should be possible to perform balloon dilation in the penis just as it is done now for renal or coronary arteries. To be able to actually expand the lumen of the arteries by arteriography and angioplasty, or to do balloon dilation of cholesterol plaque, would restore blood flow to the penis and, it is believed, open the way again for spontaneous erections. The procedure has already been described by some investigators.

This procedure is limited to a very small number of patients who have a narrowed artery (either traumatic or post-surgical) closer to the body trunk than to the penis. A cannula—or tube—is placed in the artery through the area that is narrowed. Then a balloon is filled. As the balloon is filled, the walls of the artery are stretched open. This procedure is done for coronary artery disease now and it does work; whether or not the artery closes up again is another problem. Unfortunately, I don't think this means much yet for treatment of erectile dysfunction for the following reasons:

1) It is fairly complicated and difficult to tell who is a good candidate for getting an arteriogram. That is a considerable procedure. The number of patients who will respond to this appears to be small—almost infinitesimal. The risk of complications is greater than any possible risks of injecting one's penis every time one wants to have sex.

2) Inflow of blood into the penis is only one of the factors influencing the erection. Penile tissue must be healthy to trap blood in the penis and keep it from going out. Thus, if a patient

has diffuse atherosclerosis, he will have decreased arterial inflow. In addition, the walls of the penis may not be as healthy or elastic and therefore they will not expand and will not trap the blood in the penis. (With an injection, you also impact the penile tissue, in addition to increasing the inflow. In angioplasty, you increase inflow only.)

Medications

What is fascinating is that erections used to be considered a mechanical problem. Now, they are becoming more and more a biochemical problem, as are many other medical problems. The field of impotence treatment is shifting toward the biochemical/pharmacological disease category, rather than being considered a mechanical disease. Thus, when the chemical balance is right, the erection works.

That doesn't mean an erection is simple. It is complicated and multifactorial. There are several different chemicals involved, along with the elasticity of the penis.

There are four ways of delivering medications to the area of the penis: One is by injection; the second is by mouth—with a pill; the third is with a patch on the skin, and the fourth is through the meatus (hole) of the penis through the urethra.

Problems with the patch: Any medication you put on the patch gets absorbed in the skin. The skin has a healthy drainage of veins, which take the medication into the main circulation where it is carried to the right side of the heart, which then pumps the medication to the lung, back to the left side of the heart, then to the liver and the organs. By that time, whatever medication you put on the patch has been absorbed and broken down unless it has been given in such huge doses as to produce side effects, such as dizziness, because these medications are vasodilators. Just because the patch is on a certain spot does not mean the medication is going right into that spot. And just because you take something, that doesn't mean you're going to absorb it. Again, you have to look at every step rigorously.

Incidentally, a patch could be placed on your shoulder; you don't have to put it on your penis.

Another problem with the patch is the fact that the lining—or fascia—of the penis that surrounds the corpus cavernosum is very thick. It is watertight. That is why no blood leaks out of it when you get an erection. So how can a medication possibly diffuse that way? Some of it may get in through some of the veins that drain the blood from the penis, but those veins *drain* blood, so the blood is going the wrong way. This certainly limits the effectiveness of the patch.

Problems with the pill: Medication taken in a pill form would get absorbed in the gastrointestinal tract. Again, like the patch, it would get into circulation and to the liver, where it gets broken down before reaching the penis.

Problems with putting medication through the urethra: We know there are tiny veins that connect the urethra to the rest of the surrounding tissues of the penis, but these are very small. Some doctors advocate using a swab to place medication in the penis. Patients who have tried this report that erections are not as good as with the injection method. However, possibly by increasing the dose of medication delivered in the urethra, enough will eventually get into the penile corpora and improve erectile response.

So that leaves the injection method as the best route at the present time. Why is it so satisfactory? Because you can give a very tiny dose that is delivered right to the affected area; also, the medication is in such a small quantity that even if it should leak out of the penis and not be broken down locally, it will do no harm because it is like a drop in the bucket of the individual's entire system.

The needle is safer and healthier for a patient than something given by mouth, or through a patch, or transurethrally. Therefore, it comes down to a matter of changing the way one looks at the needle. It is more efficacious, safer—and painless.

My impression is that for at least the next 10 years injections will remain the treatment of choice. We will, of course, be looking at different drugs. We will be looking at automatic injecting devices where you just push a button. These may be prefilled and disposable. You will be able to buy a kit at the drugstore and throw it out after you use it. It will be good to have these devices, because you can inject only once, so drug addicts can't find those needles and reuse them. You have only to make sure to recap them so no one else can be harmed with the needle, but you won't have to worry about disposal.

I think we will see some of these new drugs approved by the FDA for this use for impotence. Some of these medications may be in different forms, presented in different ways, in smaller doses. The future lies in pharmacological erections.

17

Conclusion

There is a saying, "The more you know, the luckier you become." We're all lucky to be living in the 1990s. Whereas only five years ago few options existed for the millions of men who could no longer get spontaneous, rigid erections, today's options include vacuum devices, hormone replacement, pharmacotherapy (injection therapy), implants, and surgical revascularization (arterio-venous bypass).

This book can serve as a guide to making, or helping someone else make, an educated decision about potency treatment. The choices are here right now. The options are better than they have ever been before. The future looks even more promising.

If you or your mate take the quiz at the end of this book and you believe your problem might be physical, I recommend that you contact an erectile dysfunction specialist. (A list may be found in Appendix C.)

When a man comes out of the closet—so to speak—and complains that he has a problem with erections, a doctor gets only one or two opportunities with him. If after two visits he hasn't found something that is effective and acceptable, that's it.

That man will probably never see another doctor about this problem again.

So if the opportunity to support a man in being treated is missed, if we don't make it possible for him to have erections and good sex, that's it. The opportunity is gone.

That is why I feel a man should go to a specialist from the start. Go to someone who has expertise in erectile dysfunction. That expert will do all the basic tests and it is cheaper and faster to bypass a whole series of doctors. Also, a specialist who deals with a lot of erection problems can pick up on a psychological problem right away and a lot of unnecessary tests can be avoided. You, the patient, are not so likely to get discouraged.

Above all, the important thing to keep in mind is that men no longer have to suffer from erectile dysfunction in silence, no longer have to see their intimate relationships limited or destroyed by impotence problems, no longer have to miss out on a life enriched by exhilarating and loving sex. Impotence can be treated—safely and effectively. That should be a welcome and heartening message for untold numbers of men—and for those who share their lives.

APPENDIX A

Self Quiz

No longer do we treat a man with psychological counseling for two or more years first, and then find out that he should have been treated physically. If someone has an erection problem, the first thing we do is rule out a physical problem. If everything is fine physically, then we refer the patient to a therapist. Of course, if there is a physical abnormality, that is looked into further and treatment options are offered. This thinking is the complete opposite of that of the 1960s when experts believed erection problems fell strictly within the purview of psychotherapy.

Still, most men continue to think their problems are mental and they go along hoping that they will disappear by themselves. This is why most men wait at least two years before seeking treatment.

HOW DO YOU KNOW IF YOU SHOULD SEE A SPECIALIST?

The average length of time from when an erection begins to falter to when a patient consults a doctor is two to three years. A great many men spend a lot of time thinking about their faltering sexual ability, but there is a major resistance to seeking medical advice. Part of the problem is lack of information. The quiz that follows offers a way to actually engage and act on the problem.

History taking is the most important aspect of evaluating and diagnosing erectile dysfunction. The following quiz covers some of the questions doctors ask for their records and to help in their evaluation. An explanation of these questions and what they mean to someone with potency problems follows the scoring section.

When taking this quiz, keep in mind that evaluation for erectile failure is not easy and straightforward. This quiz does not replace a visit to a specialist, nor is it intended to replace a medical consultation in making a decision as to the etiology of the problem or some of the possible treatment options. Nevertheless, if done honestly and completely, the quiz can convey a sense of whether or not an erectile problem is physical or mental. (Keep in mind that well over 80% of all impotence is physically caused.) The good news is that when a physical cause is diagnosed, there exist today safe, inexpensive and easy treatment options in the form of pharmacotherapy that were not available just 10 years ago.

Use this quiz to start thinking about the problem in a systematic, organized fashion so that there is less resistance to seeking treatment, if necessary. By completing this quiz, you will gain some insight into the problem. Circle the appropriate number and then add the Yes column replies.

SELF QUIZ

A. PERSONAL HISTORY

	YES	NO
1. Are you over 35?	1	0
2. Do you have a feeling of intimacy with your sexual partner?	1	0
3. Is your emotional relationship with your sexual partner a good one?	1	0
4. Do you find your sexual partner attractive?	1	0
5. Are your erections as good as they were at the very start of the relationship? As they have been throughout the relationship?	1	0
6. Is this the first time you have experienced erection problems?	1	0
7. Are you currently happy with work relationships?	1	0
8. Are you currently happy with home relationships?	1	0
TOTAL		

B. MEDICAL HISTORY

	YES	NO
1. Are you over 50?	1	0
2. Do you have any illness or medical condition?	1	0
3. Do you have any history of diabetes mellitus?	1	0
4. Have you noticed a change in the shape of your erect penis?	1	0
5 Has a doctor ever diagnosed high blood pressure?	1	0
6. Do you have any heart disease, history of stroke, or vascular disease?	1	0
7. Do you have any kidney disease, or history of alcoholism?	1	0
8. Do you take antihypertensive medications?	1	0
9. Have you recently had any pelvic surgery?	1	0
10. Have you received any radiation therapy to the pelvic area?	1	0
11. Have you received any chemotherapy?	1	0
12. Do you have cancer of the prostate or any cancers that are localized in the pelvic area?	1	0
13. Do you have sexual fantasies often?	1	0
14. Do you have a history of smoking?	1	0
15. Do you use recreational drugs?	1	0
16. Do you drink more than four ounces of alcohol daily?	1	0
TOTAL		

C. ERECTILE HISTORY

	YES	NO
1. Did problems begin gradually?	1	0
2. Can you presently get a partial erection?	1	0
3. Has the quality of morning and night-time erections decreased?	1	0

C. ERECTILE HISTORY *(continued)*

	YES	NO
4. Are your erections influenced by different partners?	1	0
5. Is there a change in penis sensitivity?	1	0
7. Does penetration ability vary with position?	1	0
8. Does erection improve when you are standing?	1	0
9. If you do get an erection, are you unable to maintain it?	1	0
10. Do you often ejaculate with a soft penis?	1	0
11. Does it take more time now to get any kind of an erection?	1	0
12. Do you have to stuff your penis by hand into the vagina in order to penetrate?	1	0
13. Is it difficult to maintain an erection after penetration?	1	0
14. Is your erection with masturbation similar to your erection while having sex?	1	0
TOTAL		

SCORING

(Count 1 for every Yes answer; 0 for every No.)

SECTION A—PERSONAL HISTORY: A score of four or more signals a problem that is most likely physical. Three or less means a probably psychological cause.

SECTION B—MEDICAL HISTORY: A score of three or more suggests that the problem may be physical. Two or less—psychological.

SECTION C—ERECTILE HISTORY: A score of six or more indicates the problem could be physical. Four or less signals a possible psychological cause of the problem.

BREAKDOWN OF SCORING

SECTION A—PERSONAL HISTORY

Young patients (less than 35 years old) are more apt to have psychological rather than physical problems. At that age, there is little likelihood of cholesterol deposits. Even if you eat a high-fat diet, this hasn't had the time to affect the arteries yet. The aging process starts around age 50. Nonetheless, a physical cause must always be ruled out.

If no intimacy is present, then the problem is most likely to be psychological, or at least to have a psychological component. Then one has to look at other factors, including age and medical condition to get a sense of whether it could be psychological *and* physical. This gives a clue that there must be some psychological component.

If the emotional relationship is adequate with one sexual partner, then this problem with erections is, again, most likely physical. If the sexual partner is attractive, this obviously indicates that there is adequate sexual stimulus.

If erections are as good throughout a relationship as at the beginning, this indicates a low probability for a psychological problem. On the other hand, if you have problems in the beginning of a relationship, but these subside with greater intimacy, then this is more likely to be psychological.

If this is the first time that erectile dysfunction is experienced, then this is most likely to be organic, since patients with psychological problems tend to have recurrences throughout their life.

If you are happy at work and with the relationship at home, there is less likelihood of a psychological problem.

SECTION B—MEDICAL HISTORY

When a medical condition or illness is present, the problem is probably physical.

A history of diabetes indicates that the problem is physical. Diabetes has a bimodal effect in that it hits the nerves in the beginning, and then the patient goes on insulin and is being controlled. Twenty to 30 years later, the insulin-dependent diabetic develops problems associated with that disease. A 20-year history of blood sugars that are not always well controlled promotes cholesterol deposits. These slowly obstruct the arteries. It is at that point that diabetics will have marked decrease in blood flow in the arteries of the penis and the problem with erections becomes irreversible. At first, the problem will most likely be with the nerves (reversible); in the long term it's the arteries (irreversible).

If there is a change in the shape of the penis, this represents a disease called Peyronie's disease, which tends to herald a physical problem.

A history of high blood pressure, heart disease, stroke, vascular disease, kidney disease, or chronic alcoholism indicates that there may be a physical cause since each of these can adversely affect erections. Hypertensive medications taken for hardening of the arteries may cause problems with erections by lowering blood pressure in the body. When systemic blood pressure is lowered, the blood pressure that goes to the penis is also decreased.

History of pelvic surgery, radiation therapy, or cancer in the pelvic area indicates that damage to the tissue of the penis and scarring of the arteries may be present. Therefore, a physical cause of the erection problem is likely.

Libido: How is your desire? Do you have a normal amount of fantasies? All men fantasize. If you have fantasized often and then suddenly stopped, or if you have fantasized a little and stopped, there has been a change in your own normal, healthy pattern of sexuality. That is what we look for in considering low hormone levels.

The libido is a correlate of testosterone level. So if you have low testosterone, your sexual desire will be down. Also, your pubic hair and beard growth slows down, so you may find that you don't need to shave as often as you once did. Also, the volume of semen goes down. Sensitivity of the penis diminishes. All these are clues that this might be a hormonal problem. Sometimes, men lose their desire to have sex because they are frustrated about their erections, so this isn't always a clear-cut issue. Was the libido lost first or was the erection? There are further clues that tell us if this could be a hormonal problem.

A history of smoking indicates that there was an insult to the cardiovascular system that can cause arterial disease. Use of recreational drugs, such as cocaine, causes spasms of the arteries, especially at the level of the coronary arteries. This can produce chest pain, for which patients often medicate themselves with nitropace, which causes problems with erections.

Heavy alcohol drinking could indicate psychological distress, because people often drink a lot when they haven't resolved issues in their lives. In a long-term alcoholic, the liver can be affected. With the liver failing, the estrogen, a natural breakdown product of testosterone, doesn't get broken down so estrogen body content increases. Breasts engorge (gynecomastia), atrophy of testes occurs, and impotence results. By this time, a man is very sick, as well. We don't see these cases often because their libido is not there due to low testosterone.

SECTION C—ERECTILE HISTORY

How is your erection now? When did it start going bad? If the problem started gradually, this indicates that it is most likely physical. If acute, it's worthwhile waiting a month before doing anything, because sometimes stressful situations resolve themselves and take care of the problem. A psychological problem would be ongoing. It would come back. Physical erectile dysfunction tends to be more of a steady worsening course without periods of real improvement. If someone has a problem at 35, is well for 10 years, and then has a problem again, that is probably psychological. But if you have a problem over the last six months, get a little bit better over vacation, then worsen again when you return home, the problem is probably physical even though it improved during vacation. It is still, overall, a gradual, downhill course.

If a partial erection is obtained, this indicates a physical problem. A patient with psychological hangups usually has no erection at all. Patients with a physical cause can often obtain a partial but insufficient erection.

Decreasing quality of morning and nighttime erections indicates a physical problem. Patients with blocked arteries often report that morning erections are much better than sexually induced erections. Men with physical erectile dysfunction can still have morning and night erections.

If someone has great sex with one partner and not another, the problem is likely to be psychological. If you masturbate without problems, but have a problem with sex in the beginning of a relationship, the problem is in the head.

When gravity is needed to supplement the erection, there is undoubtedly partial blockage of the arteries in the penis. Some men with partial blockage will report that their erections are better when they are standing, and that if they lie down, they lose their erections.

Patients with blocked arteries describe that their erections are slower to develop, and that full rigidity is never achieved. If a patient is able to obtain an erection but is not able to maintain it, then this also indicates the problem is physical.

Ejaculation with a soft penis, if this happens chronically, is a good indication that there is a physical problem with the penis. One of the first things that happens with organic erectile dysfunction is that rigidity goes down. A man loses erections before ejaculation. Erections are better when he is standing. He needs more vigorous manual stimulation in order to penetrate. Then, as they get older, men complain of premature ejaculation. (Once they enter, they are so excited they ejaculate.) They are either soft—or ready to ejaculate immediately. They are not suffering from premature ejaculation, however, but rather from decreased blood flow—vascular obstruction.

If it takes more time to obtain an erection than in the past, this indicates decrease of the blood circulation to the penis.

If the penis has to be held at the base and stuffed in order to penetrate the vagina and if it is difficult to maintain an erection after penetration, a physical problem is indicated. Men with psychological problems are happy if they just get an erection. Of course, if they can't get one, they can't penetrate. It's all or nothing with these men.

If erections with masturbation are not any better than the sexual erection, then this is definitely a sign that there is a physical problem. Masturbation is the strongest stimulation for a man to obtain an erection; therefore, it is currently believed that this is the firmest erection that can be obtained. Psychological sufferers are an unpredictable group. Some masturbate but can't maintain it. Some masturbate and ejaculate, but with a partner they are too anxious and unable to do either.

A great many men suffer mainly from unrealistic expectations. Young men think that they can go on indefinitely making love two to three times a day. Or a man in his early 40s may think his erections are "going down" because his penis droops a little bit. He calls that "softening of the penis" because it hangs down, when actually a penis will droop somewhat with age.

If onset is gradual, if you have other evidence of atherosclerotic vascular disease such as hypertension or blockage of the arteries in the legs, if you recently had pelvic surgery, if you have ejaculation with a soft penis, if you try intercourse many times and penetrate only once, your problem is probably not in your head. It is physical. On the other hand, if you try only twice and then give up, it probably is psychological.

The important thing to keep in mind is that if you are having erection problems, you should be examined by an erectile specialist. The quality of the rest of your life may depend on it.

APPENDIX B

Further Reading

1. Love, Sex, and Aging, by Edward Brecher. New York: Free Press, 1984.
2. The Potent Male, by Irwin Goldstein, M.D. & Larry Rothstein, Los Angeles: The Body Press, 1990.
3. The New Sex Therapy, by H.S. Kaplan, M.D., Ph.D. New York: Brunner/Mazel, 1974.
4. It's Not All In Your Head, by Bruce & Eileen MacKenzie. New York: E.P. Dutton, 1988.
5. Love Again, Live Again, by Steven Morganstern, M.D. & Allen Abrahams, Ph.D. Englewood Cliffs, N.J.: Prentice Hall, 1988.
6. The Sexual Self, by Avodah K. Offit, M.D. New York: Congdon & Weed, 1977.
7. Sexuality and Aging, Robert Solnick, Ed. New York: Free Press, 1978.
8. Contemporary Management of Impotence & Fertility, by Emil A. Tanagho, Thom F. Lue, & R. Dale McClure. Baltimore: Williams & Wilkins, 1988.
9. Sexual Health in Later Life, by Thomas Walz & Nancee Blum. New York: Free Press, 1987.
10. Diagnosis and Management of Impotence, by Adrian W. Zorgniotti, M.D. & Eli F. Lizza, M.D. Philadelphia: B.C. Decker, 1991.

APPENDIX C

Centers For Pharmacological Treatment of Erectile Dysfunction

Stephen M. Auerbach, M.D.
400 Newport Center Dr., Suite 501
Newport Beach, CA 92660
Phone: (714) 644-7200

Gopile H. Badlani, M.D.
Brett Mellinger, M.D.
Div. Neurourology
Long Island Jewish Medical Ctr.
New Hyde Park, NY 10042
Phone: (718) 470-7000

Richard E. Berger, M.D.
Director of Reproductive and
Sexual Medicine Clinic
Dept. of Urology, RL-10
University of Washington
1959 N.E. Pacific Street
Seattle, WA 98105
Phone: (206) 543-3640

John Boullier, M.D.
Raul Parra, M.D.
St. Louis University Hospital
3635 Vista At Grand Avenue
P.O. Box 15250

St. Louis, MO 63110-0250
Phone: (314) 577-8791

Gregory Broderick, M.D.
Fifth Floor, Silverstein Bldg.
Division of Urology
Hospital of the Univ. of
  Pennsylvania
3400 Spruce Street
Philadelphia, PA 19104
Phone: (215) 622-7331

Jeffrey Buch, M.D.
The University of Connecticut
Health Center
Division of Urology,
Dept. of Surgery
263 Farmington Avenue
Farmington, CT 06037-3955
Phone: (203) 679-3430

Troy Burns, M.D.
153 West 151st Street
Suite 150
Olathe, KS 66061
Phone: (913) 829-1501

156 MAKING LOVE AGAIN

Culley Carson, M.D.
University of North Carolina
at Chapel Hill
Campus Box 7235
Dept. of Urology
Chapel Hill, NC. 27599

Melvin J. Duckett, M.D.
Maryland Regional Impotence
Center
1104 Kenilworth Drive, Suite 406
Baltimore, MD 21204
Phone: (410) 296-6742

J. Francois Eid, M.D.
Director, Erectile Dysfunction
Unit
The New York Hospital-Cornell
Med. Ctr.
428 East 72nd Street, Suite 400
New York, NY 10021
Phone: (212) 746-5473

Irving Fishman, M.D.
Baylor College of Medicine
6624 Fannin Street, Suite 1280
Houston, TX 77030
Phone: (713) 798-5150

Jackson Fowler, M.D.
University of Mississippi
Division of Urology
2500 N. State Street
Jackson, MS 39216
Phone: (601) 984-5185

Harold A. Fuselier, M.D.
Ochsner Clinic, Dept. of Urology
1514 Jefferson Highway
New Orleans, LA 70121
Phone: (504) 838-4083

Bruce R. Gilbert, M.D., Ph.D.
900 Northern Blvd., Suite 230

Great Neck, NY 11021
Phone: (516) 487-2700

Irwin Goldstein, M.D.
New England Male Reprod.
Ctr.
University Hospital
720 Harrison Avenue
Boston, MA 02118
Phone: (617) 638-8477

Jose Gonzalez, M.D.
William Beaumont Hospital
Medical Office Building
3535 W. Mile Road, Suite
407
Royal Oak, MI 48073
Phone: (313) 551-3550

Irvin H. Hirsch, M.D.
Dept. of Urology, Rm 1112
Jefferson Medical College
1025 Walnut Street
Philadelphia, PA 19107
Phone: (215) 955-6961/6963

Nachum M. Katlowitz, M.D.
953 49th Street
Brooklyn, NY 11219
Phone: (718) 438-3475

Dean Knoll, M.D.
Center for Urological Treatment
& Research
2201 Murphy Avenue, Suite
115
Nashville, TN 37203
Phone: (615) 340-6460

Laurence A. Levine, M.D.
The University of Chicago
Section of Urology
5841 S. Maryland Avenue
Chicago, IL 60637
Phone: (312) 702-6150

Ronald W. Lewis, M.D.
Professor of Urology
Mayo Clinic
200 First Street, S.W.
Rochester, MN 55905
Phone: (507) 284-2511

Tom F. Lue, M.D.
Dept. of Urology, UCSF
533 Parnassus Avenue, U575
San Francisco, CA 94143-0736
Phone: (415) 476-8849

Michael P. O'Leary, M.D., M.P.H.
Dept. of Urology
New England Medical Center
  Hospitals
Box #269
750 Washington Street
Boston, MA 02111
Phone: (617) 956-5357

Arnold Melman, M.D.
Montefiore Medical Center
111 East 210 Street
Bronx, NY 10467
(718) 920-5402

D. Karl Montaque, M.D.
Director of the Center for Sexual
  Function
Head of Section of Prostatic
  Surgery
9500 Euclid Avenue
Cleveland, OH 44195
Phone: (216) 444-5599

John Mulcahy, M.D.
Wishard Memorial Hospital
1001 West 10th Street
Old Part-3rd Floor
Indianapolis, IN 46202
Phone: (317) 639-6671/630-6229

Thomas Mulligan, M.D.
Chief Geriatrics Med. Section (181)

Vet. Affairs Med. Center
1201 Broad Rock Blvd.
Richmond, VA 23249
Phone: (804) 230-1303

Myron Murdock, M.D.
7500 Hanover Pkwy, Suite 206
Green Belt, MD 20770
Phone: (301) 441-8900/2004

Perry Nadig, M.D.
Metropolitan Professional Building
1303 McCullough, Suite 561
San Antonio, TX 78212
Phone: (512) 227-9376

Harin Padma-Nathan, M.D.
Dept. of Urology
USC Med. Ctr.
Suite GH 5900
2025 Zonal Avenue
Los Angeles, CA 90033
Phone: (213) 224-5399

William M. Patterson, M.D.
Pres., Birmingham Res. Group,
  Inc.
6869 Fifth Avenue South
Birmingham, AL 35212
Phone: (205) 836-3594

Charles Reid, M.D.
Piedmont Research Associates
1901 S. Hawthorne Road,
  Suite 306
Winston-Salem, N.C. 27103
Phone: (919) 768-8062

Martin Resnick, M.D.
Department of Urology
Univ. Hospitals of Cleveland
2065 Adelbert Road
Cleveland, OH 44106
Phone: (216) 844-3011

Jacob Rajfer, M.D.
UCLA Medical Center
10833 LeConte Avenue
Los Angeles, CA 90024
Phone: (310) 206-8164

Johnny B. Roy, M.D.
Dept of Urology
University of Oklahoma
Health Sciences Center
P.O. Box 2690
Oklahoma, City, OK 73190
Phone: (405) 271-6900

Robert T. Segraves, M.D.
Department of Psychiatry
MetroHealth Medical Center
2500 MetroHealth Drive
Cleveland, OH 44109
Phone: (216) 459-4428

Ridwan Shabsigh, M.D.
Columbia Presb. Hospital
Department of Urology
5141 Broadway, Rm. 1-119
New York, NY 10034
Phone: (212) 305-8607

John F. Stecker, M.D.
Devine-Fiveash Urology, Ltd.
400 W. Brambelton Ave., Suite 100
Norfolk, VA 23510
Phone: (804) 628-3532

Jacques Susset, M.D.
Clinical Professor of Urology
Rhode Island Urodynamics, Inc.

100 Highland Avenue
Providence, RI 02906
Phone: (401) 331-1055

Steven Varady, M.D.
David Weinstein, M.D.
Florida Center For Impotence
114 JFK Drive
Atlantis, FL 33462
Phone: (407) 964-1607

Steven Weiner, M.D.
Boulder Medical Center
2750 Broadway
Boulder, CO 80304
Phone: (303) 440-3093

Charles White, M.D.
Coastal Clinical Research
6701 Airport Boulevard,
    Box 4
Mobile, AL 36608
Phone: (205) 639-1661

Henry A. Wise, II, M.D.
Ohio Urology
3555 Olentangy River Road,
    Suite 2050
Columbus, OH 43214
Phone: (614) 263-1876

**Eli Lizza, M.D. Adrian
    Zorgniotti, M.D.**
Urologist
33 East 74th Street
New York, NY 10021
Phone: (212) 249-3064

APPENDIX D

Support Groups

1. Impotence Anonymous, 119 S. Ruth St., Maryville, TN 37801-5746. (Chapters throughout the country. Send them a note, enclosing a stamped, self-addressed envelope.)
2. Not For Men Only, c/o Mercy Hospital and Medical Center, Stevenson Expressway at King Dr., Chicago, IL 60616. (312-567-5567 or 1-800-448-8664). For couples as well as separate groups for men and women.
3. Recovery of Male Potency (ROMP), c/o Grace Hospital, 18700 Meyers Road, Detroit, MI 48235. (1-800-TEL-ROMP outside MI; MI residents 313-927-3219). Chapters in many states.
4. Potency Restored, c/o Giulio Scarzella, M.D., 8630 Fenton St., Suite 218, Silver Spring, MD 10910. Chapters in many states.
5. The Impotence Information Center, P.O. Box 9, Dept. USA, Minneapolis, MN 55440. (1-800-843-4315). Helps people to find a support group in their area.
6. The American Association of Sex Educators, Counselors and Therapists (AASECT), 11 Dupont Circle, N.W., Suite 220, Washington, DC 20036. (202-462-1171). Offers assistance in finding a sex therapist.

Index

Ache, 93
    cause of, 57
    as side effect, 118
Admission, as first step, 25-26
Adrenal glands, tumors in as
    cause of erection
        problems, 47
Age
    patients average, 91
    and testosterone level, 63
Aging
    and arterial disease,
        66-67
    case of, 29-32
    as cause of erection
        problems, 43-44
    effects of, 114
    impotence and, 22-24
    and potency, 8
Air, injecting, 88-89, 117
Alcohol.
    as cause of erection
        problems, 42
    as depressant, 20
    and psychological

        distress, 148
Alcoholism, chronic, and
    erectile dysfunction, 147-
        148
Alcohol swab, 95-96, 119
Allen, Lloyd, 57, 121
Alpha methyl dopa, and
    erection problems, 61
Alzheimer's disease
    treatment of, 116
    and use of papaverine, 55
Angina, cocaine-induced, 41
Angiography, 80-81
Angioplasty
    assessment of, 137-138
    procedure for, 137
    as treatment for erectile
        dysfunction, 137-138
Anoxic, defined, 122
Antihistamines, and erection
    problems, 61
Antihypertensive medication
    as cause of erection
        problems, 41
    effect of on erection, 35-

36
    See also Blood pressure;
        Hypertension; Medi-
        cations
Arterial blockage
    confirmation of, 80
    and lowering cholesterol,
        129
    pharmacological erections
        as cure for, 121-122
    and timing of erection,
        121
    See also Arteries, blocked
Arterial disease, testing for,
    66-67
Arteries
    abnormal, and erection
        problems, 61
    blocked, 40-41, 108
    blocked, and gravity, 149-
        150
    blocked, and morning
        erections, 149
Arteriogenic dysfunction, 40,
    106
    See also Arteries, blocked
Arteriography, 67
Arteriovenous bypass, as
    potency treatment, 141
Atherosclerosis and
    angioplasty, 137-138
    cause of, 105
    defined, 60

diagnosis of, 76
    and smoking, 122
Atherosclerotic vascular
    disease, 16
    lack of blood in, 35

Balloon dilation
    assessment of, 137-138
    efficacy of, 137-138
    procedure for, 137
Beta blockers, 61
Bicycle seat injuries, 132
Binding, 56
Biochemical problem, erectile
    dysfunction as, 105, 138
Blood, lack of in atheroscle-
    rotic vascular disease, 35
Blood flow
    decreased, 150
    diabetes and decrease in,
        147
    Doppler test for, 75
    during erection, 34-35
    problems with, 66
    in veins, 47
Blood pressure, high, 122
    and erectile dysfunction,
        148
    and "mean systolic
        pressure," 34-35
    See also Hypertension
Blood trapping, mechanism of,
    135

Brain tumor, as cause of erection problems, 47

Breasts, engorgement of, 149

Brindley, G. S., 53-54

Calcium deposits, in penis, 36

Cancer, and erectile dysfunction, 148

Cannula, 137

Cavallini, Giorgio, 134, 134n

Cholesterol, high, 108
    cause of, 105
    and diabetes, 147
    effects of, 122
    and erectile dysfunction, 92
    and erection problems, 66

Cholesterol plaque, balloon dilation of, 137

Climax. See Orgasm

Clinical trials, need for, 124
    See also Food and Drug Administration

Closed prostate surgery, 43

Cocaine
    effect of on erection, 41
    and erectile dysfunction, 148

Colon cancer, surgery for as cause of erection problems, 60

Combined Injection and Stimulation Test, 66-71

Control, erections and, 24-25

Corpora, 102

Corpus cavernosum, 139

Coumadin, and injection testing, 67

Curvature, penile, 68, 86
    See also Peyronie's disease

Cylinders, 84-85

Detrusor muscles, 132

Detumescence, 37

Diabetes
    case of, 13-14
    as cause of erection problems, 44-45, 49-50
    and injection testing, 67
    and physical erectile problems, 147

Diabetic(s)
    decreased blood flow of, 147
    management of, 13

DICC. See Dynamic Infusion Cavernosometry-Cavernosography

Disease(s), as cause of erection problems, 44-45

Diuretics, as cause of erection problems, 41

Dizziness, as side effect, 118,

138-139
Doppler Ultrasound Test
(DUPLEX), 75-76
Drawing needle, 96
Drinking, and erection prob-
lems, 61
See also Alcohol
Drugs
background on, 53-58
as cause of erection
problems, 41
recreational, 148
See also Medication(s)
DUPLEX, 75-76, 93, 106
See also Doppler Ultra-
sound Test
Dynamic Infusion
Cavernosometry-
Cavernosography
(DICC), 79-80

Ejaculation
and erection, 59
premature, 150
retrograde, 41
with soft penis, 64-65,
150
Erectile dysfunction (ED), 62-
63
admission of, as first step,
25-26
as branch of urology, 2
as biochemical problem,

105, 138
centers for pharmological
158
as first symptom, 45
and injection therapy, 4
pharmological approach
to, 106
physical basis for, 147-
149
physical vs. psychologi-
cal, 149
psychogenic, 18, 65, 78
psychological basis for,
147
questions concerning
treatment
for, 115-127
specialists in treatment of,
142, 155-158
support groups for, 159
as symptom, 74
vascular, 105
Erectile history, 145-146
scoring, 149-151
Erection(s)
and antihypertension
medication, 35-36
and control, 24-25
decrease in strength of,
34
duration of pharmacologi-
cal, 57
and ejaculation, 59

enhancement of by stimu-
    lation, 67
and hormone level, 35
how it happens, 33-37
maintenance of, 121
measuring rigidity of, 79
medically-induced, 54
medical questions con-
    cerning, 64-66
morning, 65, 149
nighttime, 65, 76-78, 149
and orgasm, 58
physical problems with,
    13
prolonged, 119,
prolonged, and psycho-
    genic problems, 8
prolonged, as side effect,
    56-57
psychological factors for,
    62-63
psychogenic problems
    with, 33-34
quality of, 65
reflex, 33
rigid phase of, 35
self-evaluation of, 69
as symbol of manhood, 40
use of medications to
    control, 15-16
Erection problems
    abnormal arteries and, 61
    causes of, 39-51

effect of medications on,
    61
    See also Erectile dysfunc-
        tion
Estrogen
    as breakdown product, 42
    and libido, 47
    and liver function, 148-
        149
Exercise
    clothing for, 132
    and potency, 130-131
External vacuum tumescence,
    83

Fascia, of penis, 139
Fibrosis, as side effect, 56
Food and Drug Administration
    (FDA)
    approval of erection-
        inducing medications,
        54, 140
    on injection medications,
        123-124
Foreplay, 102
    and erection, 57
    value of, and erection,
        121
Foreskin, 96-97

Glucose levels, high, 44
Glucotrol, 14
Gonorrhea, 49

Gravity, and blocked arteries, 149-150

Gynecomastia, 149

Hair, growth of, and testosterone level, 148

HDLs, 130

Headache, as side effect, 118

Heart disease, and erectile dysfunction, 148

High-fat diet, and erection problems, 129-130

High serum-cholesterol levels, and erection problems, 129-130

See also Cholesterol, high

History taking

importance of detailed, 59-60, 143-144

value of, 78-79

Homosexual encounters, 62

Hormone level

and erection, 35

and libido, 148

of thyroid gland, 48

Hormone replacement, 83

as potency treatment, 141

Hormones

blood test for, 70

and causes of erection problems, 45-46

Hospital of Adria (Venetto, Italy), 134

Hypertension, 107

effect of medications for, 148

and injection testing, 67

as risk factor, 60

treatment for reducing, 130

See also Blood pressure, high

Implant(s)

as potency treatment, 141

recommendations for, 57

Impotence

and aging, 22-24

biochemical/pharmacological aspect of, 138

causes of, 2, 50-51

and defects in nitrous oxide system, 135

population at risk for, 39-40

and prostatectomy, 60

treatment for, 142

warning signals of, 50-51

Inderal, and erection problems, 61

Injecting needle, 96

Injection(s)

advantage of, 108, 109

background on, 17-18

contraindications to, 58

and foreplay, 57

frequency of, 120
improvement in methods
    of, 140
inadequate response to,
    123
limitations of, 58
number of, 57
and pain, 120
as painless, 89
sexual life with, 114
success rate of, 120
timing of, 122-123
too frequent, 123
trial, 90-91
use of, 86-87
weaning off, 21
women's reaction to,
    112-114
Injection method, as satisfac-
    tory,139-140
Injection pharmacotherapy,
    centers for, 7
Injection therapy, 2-4
    cases of, 105-109
    cost of, 91
    for erectile dysfunction, 4
        and FDA, 124
    as potency treatment, 141
    reasons for, 83-94
Institute of Psychiatry (London), 53
Insulin, and potency difficul-
    ties, 41

Insurance, coverage
    oferectionproblems, 124
Intimacy
    implications of lack of,
        147
    importance of, 20
    need for, 103, 127
    and potency, 7-8
    See also Romance
Intra-penile pressure, 36

Jock strap, use of, 132
*Journal of the American
    Medical Association*, 39
Journal of Urology, The, 54,
    133n, 134n, 136n

Kidney disease, and erectile
    dysfunction, 148

Lactic acid, formation of, 123
LDLs, 130
Lead poisoning, as cause of
    erection problems, 48
Leriche's syndrome, 6
Libido
    defined, 42, 63
    effect of alcohol on, 42
    and hormone levels, 148
Linsidomine chlorhydrate,
    136, 136n
Liver, effect of alcohol on,
    148-149
Liver enzymes, increase in,

118
Lumen, 102, 119
   arterial, dilation of, 53,
      137
   obstruction of, 60

Manual dexterity, poor, as
   contraindication to
      injection, 58, 115
Masters and Johnson, 2
Masturbation, 59, 90
   and injection stimulation,
      68-69
   and psychological erectile
   dysfunction, 149
   as strongest stimulation,
      150
Meatus, 138
Medical history, 60-61, 145
   scoring, 147-149
Medication(s)
   cost of, 120
   as enhancement, 106
   for erectile dysfunction,
      138-140
   for hypertension, 148
   influence of, on erectile
      dysfunction, 61
   "off-label" use of, 54-55
   oral, 133-135
   safety of, 116-117
   side effects from, 118
   temperature of, 103

   ways of delivering, 138-
      140
   See also Antihypertensive
      medication
Memorial Sloan-Kettering
   Cancer Center, 11
Minoxicil, research on, 134,
   134n
Mood swings, as symptom of
   multiple sclerosis, 49
Morales, Alvaro, 133, 133n
Morning erections, 65
   and blocked arteries, 149
Multiple sclerosis
   as cause of erectile
      problems, 44, 45, 48-
      49
   treatment of, 116
   and use of papaverine, 55
Mumps, as cause of erection
   problems, 45
Muscle relaxation, and nitric
   oxide, 34

N. Y. U. School of Medicine,
   54
Needle(s), 102
   dangers from use of, 119-
      120
   drawing, 96
   fineness of, 87
   injecting, 96
   safety of, 140

size of, 68
29g., 96n
use of new, 119
Nerve conduction
studies on, 67
test for, 5-6
Nerves, as cause of erection
problems, 48-50
Neurogenically impaired
patients,
treatment of, 134
*New England Journal of
Medicine*, 39, 135n
New York Hospital-Cornell
Medical Center, The, 4
Pharmacological Erection
Program of, 59
serum-cholestrol study of,
129
Night test, 27
See also Nocturnal test;
Sleep test
Nighttime erections, decreas-
ing, 149
Nighttime study sleep test, 40
Nitric oxide, 105, 135-136,
135n, 136n
and muscle relaxation, 34
Nitroglycerine, research on,
134,134n
Nitropace, 148
Noctural erections, 76-78
Nocturnal penile tumescence

studies, 67
Nocturnal testing, 5
See also Night test; Sleep
test
Nodules, formation of as side
effect, 56

Open prostate surgery, 43
Oral medications, 133-135
Orgasm, 65-66
and erection, 58
and injections, 122
Osbon Erec Aid Vacuum, 108
Overweight, and erectile
dysfunction, 126, 130
Oxytocin, research on, 134

Papaverine
cost of, 56, 120
in DICC test, 80
discovery of, 2
dosage of, 57, 116
FDA on, 123-124
first use of, 53
in mixture, 32
phentolamine as comple-
ment to, 55
safety of, 116
side effects of, 116, 118
stability of, 57, 58
use of, 116
Papaverine hydrochloride, 55
Papaverine/phentolamine

mixture, 107
response to, 93
speed of, 121
stability of, 121
temperature of, 103
Paraplegic, and response to
    papaverine, 123
Parkinson's disease, as cause
    of erection problems, 44
Partner, assistance of, 125-
    126
Patch(es)
    placement of, 139
    problems with, 138-139
    use of, 134-135
Pelvic surgery, and erectile
    dysfunction, 148
Penile blood pressure tests, 67
Penile fibrosis, 36
    See also Scarring
Penile implant
    and injection therapy, 67
    recommendation for, 94
    See also Implant(s);
        Penile prosthesis
Penile injections
    advantage of, 67-68
    common worries concern-
        ing, 88-94
    myths about, 125
    psychological aspects of,
        69-70
Penile prosthesis, 31, 83, 84-

86
    See also Implant(s);
        Penile implant
Penile pulses, testing of, 5
Penile shaft, 36
    Penis and angioplasty,
        137-138
    balloon dilation of, 137-
        138
    care of, 131-132
    curvature of, 43
    and ejaculation, 64-65
    fracture of, 131
    girth of, 78, 79
    shape of, 64
    soft, 105
    softening of, 150
    veno-occlusive mecha-
        nism of, 64
Persantine, and injection
    testing, 67
Personal history, 144
    scoring, 146-147
Peyronie's disease, 36, 37, 47,
    64, 148
    as cause of erection
        problems, 43
    symptoms of, 117-118
PGE1, 93, 108
    benefits of, 136
    cost of, 120
    dosage of, 57, 117
    and nitric oxide levels,

136
side effects of, 56-57, 118
speed of, 121
stability of, 58, 121
use of, 116
See also Prostaglandin E1
Pharmacological Erection
Program (PEP), 4, 86-87
frequency of need for, 91
Pharmacological injections,
candidates for, 115
Pharmacotherapy, as potency
treatment, 141
Phenoxybenzamine, action of,
55
Phentolamine
as complement to papav-
erine, 55
cost of, 56, 120
in DICC test, 80
discovery of, 2
dosage of, 116
FDA on, 123
in mixture, 32
research on, 53
safety of, 116
side effects of, 116, 118
in test, 66
use of, 116
Physical erectile dysfunction,
symptoms of, 150
Physical exam, 66
Physician's Desk Reference,

124
Pill, problems with, 139
Pituitary adenoma, 47
Plaque
balloon dilation of, 137
development of, 117
Potency
aging and, 8
as flagging with advanc-
ing years, 43-44
help for faltering, 29
insulin, and difficulties
with, 41
intimacy and, 7-8
women's attitude toward,
8-9
workup for, 59-71
Potency problems, prevention
of, 129-132
Potency treatment
demystification of, 12-13
methods of, 141
for spinal cord injuries, 15
Premature ejaculation, 150
Priapism
defined, 17, 49, 118
as side effect, 56
Procedures, invasive, reliance
on, 59-60
Prolonged erection, 119
danger of, 122-123
and psychological prob-
lems, 8

Prostaglandin E1 (PGE1), 106
  cost of,   56
  discovery of, 2
  FDA on, 123
  in mixture, 32
  safety of, 116-117
  temperature of, 103
  in test, 66
  uses of, 55-56
  See also PGE1
Prostate, transurethral resection of, 30
Prostate cancer
  diagnosis of, 39-40
  surgery for, 43
Prostatectomy, radical, 11
  and impotence, 60
Prosthesis, 31
  inflatable, 84
  See also Implant(s);
    Penile prosthesis
Psychogenic erectile dysfunction, 78
Psychogenic problems and
  erections, 33-34
  and prolonged erections,
  8
Psychogenic stimuli, physical
  reflex to, 33-34
Psychological erectile
  dysfunction, symptoms of,
  150, 151
Psychotherapy, and erection

problems, 143
Pump, 84-85
Px3. *See* Prostaglandin E 1

Queens University (Kingston,
  Ontario), 133

Radiation therapy
  as cause of erection
    problems, 43, 48, 60
  and erectile dysfunction,
    148
Radical prostatectomy, 11
  and impotence, 60
Rajfer, Jacob, 135, 135n
Reflex arc, 33
Reflex erection, 33
Reflex loop, 33
Regitine, 53, 55
  See also Phentolamine
Relaxation
  importance of, 24-25,
    107-108
  of muscles, 34
Reluctance, man's, 19-22
REM sleep, and nocturnal
  erections, 76-77
Reserpine, and erection
  problems, 61
Reservoir, 84-85
Retrograde ejaculation, 41
Revascularization, surgical,
  83, 141

Rigiscan, 79
Rings, use of, 108
Romance, 111-114
   and potency, 7-8
   See also Intimacy

Saline solution, in DICC test,
   80
Scarring
   occurrence of, 86
   of penis, 36
   as side effect, 56
   and too frequent injec-
      tions, 123
   See also Penile fibrosis
Scar tissue, confirmation of,
   80
Schenk, Michael, 86
Sciatic nerve, pinched, 49
Scoring, 146
   breakdown of, 146-147
Scott, Brantley, 84
Self-injection, 1
   costs of, 56
   how to, 95-103
   pharmacological, 83
   procedure for, 95, 98-101
   timing of, 95
   See also Injection therapy
Self-quiz, 143-151
Semen
   volume of, 65-66
   volume of, and testoster-

one level, 148
Sex
   disinterest in, 23
   interest in, and aging, 22-
      23
Sex therapy, 83, 106
   and injections, 91
Sickle cell disease, 115
   as contraindication to
      injection therapy, 58
Side effects
   categories of, 117
   of medication, 117-118
   of patch, 138-139
   potential, 56-57
   of steroids, 130
Sleep labs, 78
Sleep test, 21, 76-79
   See also Nocturnal test
Smoking, 108
   and atherosclerosis, 122
   as cause of erection
      problems, 42
   cessation of, 126
   and erectile dysfunction,
      61, 92, 148
   and erectile function, 58
   as risk factor, 12
Social history, 61-63
Spinal-cord injuries
   as cause for erection
      problems, 44
   potency treatment for, 15

and response to injections, 123
Steroids, side effects of, 130
Stief, C. G., 136n
Stimulation
  and erection enhancement, 67
  for trial injections, 90-91
Stroke
  and erectile dysfunction, 148
  as risk factor, 60
Support groups, 159
Surgery, as cause of erection problems, 43
Surgical revasculation, 83
  as potency treatment, 141
Swab, use of, 139
  See also Alcohol swab
Syringes, prefilled, 87, 90, 95

Testes, atrophy of, 149
Testicles, effects of mumps on, 45-46
Testing, second visit, 73-74
Test injection, initial, 26-27
Testosterone
  and estrogen, 42
  injections of, 46
  and libido, 63
Testosterone level
  and age, 63
  and libido, 148

testing of, 5, 46
Testosterone replacement, 63
Thyroid gland, hormone level of, and erection problems, 48
Tumors, as causes of erection problems, 47
Tunica albuginea, 102, 131

Ultrex-Plus (American Medical Systems), 84-86, 85
University of Oklahoma College of Pharmacy, 57, 121
Urethra
  injection of, 88, 97, 119
  medicating through, 139

Vacuum devices, as potency treatment, 141
Vascular disease, and erectile dysfunction, 148
Vascular erectile dysfunction, diagnosis of, 105
Vascularity, confirmation of abnormal, 80
Vascular obstruction, and ejaculation, 150
Vasodilator, PGE1 as, 55-56
Vein problems, as cause of erection problems, 47
Venogenic veins, 47
Venous leakage, confirmation

of, 80
Virag, Ronald, 53
Vision, poor, as
    contraindication for
      injection, 58, 115
Voiding dysfunctions, 48

Wall Street Journal, The, 16

Wyndaele, J., 54

X-rays, in DICC test, 79-80

Yacon, 133
    See also Yohimbine
Yohimbine, 92, 133, 133n

Zorgniotti, Adrian, 54